The Essential Oils

and

Aromatherapy

Handbook

by Rashelle Johnson

<u>Disclaimer:</u>

Dedication:

This book is dedicated to my family and friends, on whom I'm constantly testing out new products and essential oil blends. Thanks for being such good sports guys. I couldn't do this without you.

Contents

Introduction

The use of essential oils and aromatherapy to treat ailments and illnesses predates modern medicine by thousands of years. While I would never advocate completely eschewing modern medicine in favor of using essential oils, I do believe they can be used to effectively treat or ease the effect of some ailments. In this day and age, we're too quick to turn to the expensive medicines pushed by the big pharmaceutical companies when there may be other more holistic approaches we could try.

The term *Western medicine* refers to the use of doctors, hospitals, surgery and expensive medications to treat ailments. This is option most people turn to first when they're sick or don't feel good. Some people run to the doctor at the first sign of a problem and are prescribed a wide range of medications to cure anything and everything that's wrong with them.

The problem with this approach is that it relies on bombarding the body with a constant barrage of chemicals that it doesn't recognize. You end up treating one problem while creating others. It isn't uncommon to find people who are taking medication to treat side-effects caused by other medications. Over time, the chemical balance of your body changes and the problems you're having either intensify or new problems pop up.

It creates a never-ending cycle of medication that's great for the big pharmaceutical companies, but bad for your body— and your pocketbook.

Eastern medicine refers to time-tested techniques for treating ailments that don't require modern medicine. Eastern medicine includes acupuncture, aromatherapy and the use of herbs and essential oils to treat ailments naturally.

Essential oils have largely been ignored in modern medicine, but are experiencing something of a revival by those seeking ulterior treatments to those offered up by Western doctors. A holistic approach to health and wellness is sometimes all that's needed to cure minor illnesses and ailments.

Plant Oil Safety

Essential oils and other plant oils are without a doubt a wonderful and holistic way to enhance your physical and mental well-being. They have been shown to help people ease certain ailments and are capable of many, many things.

That said, they should never be used in lieu of medical treatment of serious illness, injuries or ailments.

There's a small, but very vocal group of people out there claiming they can cure anything and everything through holistic medicine and use of essential oils. While essential oils can be part of a treatment regimen, you do not want to bet your life solely on holistic treatment. Always, and I mean always, consult a doctor before undergoing a holistic treatment regimen and be sure to discuss any health concerns you have with your doctor prior to starting treatment.

For serious injuries and ailments, you may be able to undergo holistic treatment at the same time you're being medically treated. This is a decision you have to make with your doctor and your holistic practitioner.

If your holistic practitioner is pushing you to stop medical treatment for a serious injury or ailment, you need to consider the possible implications of stopping the treatment. If you're under a doctor's care, always inform the doctor before stopping medical treatment or starting holistic treatment. There may be concerns you aren't aware of.

Always, and I mean always, consult with your doctor before using essential oils. This is especially important if you're pregnant or have health issues.

Be aware that plant oils are the powerful essences of the plants they're derived from. They may interact negatively with prescription drugs you're currently taking. Always consult with a medical professional before starting to use plant oils. This is especially important if you're currently taking medication to treat an illness or chronic condition.

What is Aromatherapy?

Aromatherapy is the use of plant oils to promote physical and psychological well-being and health. The oils derived from plants have a number of healing properties that can be used to help treat a number of illnesses and ailments. Aromatherapy can be used to relax the mind, body and soul, while restoring balance and harmony both spiritually and physically.

Essential oils play a key role in the world of aromatherapy, as they're the essence of the plants they're taken from. The use of these oils is both an art form and a science, as a skilled practitioner can use aromatherapy techniques as both a preemptive measure to stop ailments before they occur and as a form of treatment for many chronic and acute diseases.

While I would never suggest using aromatherapy as the only line of defense against a disease that's ravaging one's body, there are a number of people out there who swear by essential oils and claim they were able to treat and cure a number of diseases and illnesses through careful use of essential oils and aromatherapy. What I suggest is using these oils *in addition to* the Western medicine, at least at first. You may find your doctor is eventually able to wean you off the medications you've grown accustomed to. This is a decision that should be made under the supervision of a medical professional and isn't something you should do on your own.

Aromatherapy is a holistic approach that seeks to treat and prevent health problems in a natural manner. The human body has a remarkable ability to heal itself, and aromatherapy seeks to capitalize on that ability by enhancing the body's natural capabilities.

While one could reasonably surmise aromatherapy involves only inhaling the scent of plant oils, it also encompasses other methods of applying oils to the body. Physical application and inhalation of the aromas of plant oils are both important methods of delivery that fall under the blanket term aromatherapy.

Tips for Those New to the World of Aromatherapy

Aromatherapy can be confusing to those seeking to begin their journey into the realm of plant oils. You have to be willing to accept that modern medicine isn't always the only answer to your woes. You have to enter your journey with an open mind and be ready for new and exciting experiences.

Beginning your journey is an exciting time, but there are pitfalls you need to watch out for. There are people and companies out there looking to take advantage of those who don't have much knowledge. The following tips will help ease your transition into the world of aromatherapy:

1. Don't believe everything you hear.

There's a lot of misinformation out there regarding essential oils and aromatherapy. Some people will say it doesn't work. Some will make exaggerated claims, saying it cures anything and everything. The truth lies somewhere in the middle. Use common sense and don't go in expecting miracles and you'll be pleased with the results.

Believing everything you hear can be downright dangerous.

I've seen websites that claim essential oils can cure everything from cancer to sexually transmitted diseases. Most of the sites have since been taken down, but someone who read that and believed it could potentially do irreparable harm by stopping treatment and trying to make the switch to essential oils. Again, if you see a claim that seems too good to be true, it probably is. Don't fall for exaggerated claims and make all treatment decisions in concordance with your doctor's recommendations, not against what your doctor recommends.

2.   Research. Research. Research.

Beginners tend to want to buy a bunch of different essential oils and start rubbing them all over their bodies in a misguided attempt to cure anything and everything they have wrong. This is the wrong approach. It will cost you a lot of money and leave you disappointed in the end. It might even do you more harm than good.

Carefully research the oils you're interested in and carefully research the companies you're thinking about buying them from. You want the best oils for your body, and you need to make sure you're getting them from reputable companies with a proven track record. Essential oils are largely unregulated and quality can vary widely. Make sure you pay close attention to what you're buying, as some suppliers use trickery and smoke and mirrors to make you think you're buying essential oils when the truth is you're getting something entirely different.

3.   Take the time to find the right combination of oils for your body.

No two human bodies are the same.

We all have a different balance of chemicals and hormones in our body. Aromatherapy seeks to realign and harmonize this balance. Since we're all different, it stands to reason that we need to find the right formula of essential oils for our body type and chemical composition. What works great for one person may not work for another. Conditions one body thrives under may not be conducive to good health for another body.

A slow, calculated approach works best. It helps to remember that while essential oils are natural, they are powerful and your body is going to need time to adjust to them. Start slow and try an oil or two at a time, taking careful note of how your body reacts to them. Slowly bring your body into alignment and figure out the dosages and essential oils that work best for you.

4. Know what you're buying.

Make sure you only buy 100% pure therapeutic grade essential oils if you plan on using them for aromatherapy. Anything less isn't acceptable. Good essential oils aren't cheap. Go too cheap and you run the risk of buying essential oil that's mixed with synthetic chemicals or has been removed from the plant via a method that damages the oil and leaves trace amounts of harmful chemicals behind.

Perfume oils are not the same as essential oils. All you get with perfume oils is a good smell. They don't work for aromatherapy and don't have the same natural agents that essential oils have.

All essential oils are not made the same. The quality of the oil depends largely on the quality of the plant they're derived form. There are different varieties of plants that can be used to make oils that carry the same name. An example of this is Lavender oil. It can come from a number of different varieties of lavender plant. If you find one you like and it seems to work well, pay close attention to the botanical name of the plant the oil is taken from. The botanical name is the scientific name of the plant. One plant used to make lavender oil is Lavandula angustifolia.

5. Avoid containers that use rubber.

Essential oils are strong enough to eat through rubber and will eventually melt rubber away. This will ruin your essential oil because the chemicals in the rubber will combine with your oil to create new harmful compounds instead of the healthy compounds they normally contain.

For this reason, you should only use glass containers to store your essential oils in. While rubber droppers are nice when it comes time to measure out your oil, don't store your oil in a container that has a rubber dropper attached to it.

6. All essential oils aren't made from organically-grown plants.

The way the plants an essential oil is made from are grown can compromise the integrity of the oil. If a crop is pummeled with chemical fertilizers, herbicides and pesticides before it's harvested, some of those chemicals can make their way into your essential oils. Sure, it'll only be there in trace amounts, but I'd much rather have no synthetic chemicals in my essential oil than just a little bit.

7. Heed all safety warnings before you start using an oil.

Essential oils need to be used with caution. Make sure you do your due diligence before using a new oil. Consult with your physician and with an aromatherapy expert before attempting to treat any condition you have through aromatherapy. Always test new oils by using only a small amount at first and wait to see if there's an adverse reaction. If your body reacts adversely, discontinue use immediately.

If you are pregnant, always consult a physician before using essential oils. Some oils that are perfectly safe when you aren't pregnant may pose a significant risk to your unborn fetus.

8. Keep your essential oils away from children.

Kids love essential oils because they smell fantastic. What children often don't realize is that essential oils are a lot stronger than they smell. Letting a kid play around with essential oils is a recipe for disaster.

While there are some essential oils generally considered safe for use with children, they should only be used in small amounts and under adult supervision. Store your essential oils where your kids can't get to them so there aren't any accidents.

9. Consumption of essential oils is to be avoided unless prescribed by a doctor.

Essential oils can pose a health hazard if consumed. You should not eat or otherwise ingest essential oils on their own or as part of a blend with carrier oils or any other substance unless they've been prescribed by a professional practitioner. Essential oils can be toxic to the liver and other internal organs when ingested.

10. Avoid letting your essential oils come into contact with anything other than glass.

While some plastics are safe to keep essential oils in, a good rule of thumb is to only store your oils in glass containers. You need to avoid letting them come in contact with all other storage mediums. Metal is especially bad, as it can react with certain essential oils and permanently change the chemical composition.

What Are Essential Oils?

Essential oils are natural oils extracted from plant matter through a distillation process. They are known by a number of names, including volatile oils and ethereal oils. They are also referred to as the "oil of" or "essence of" the particular plant they were derived from.

In addition to medicinal use, essential oils are used to naturally scent a number of products on the market today. From perfumes to household cleaning products, essential oils provide a wide array of scents ranging from pine trees to citrus and everything in-between. Essential oils don't just smell good, they're even added to some food products and drinks to add flavor.

Essential oils are extracted from the plants that hold them using a number of methods. The method of extraction and the ability of the person or machine doing the extraction largely determine the quality of the oil. The chemical composure of essential oils can be altered during the extraction process, rendering the oil useless for the desired intent and purpose.

Distillation is one of the extraction methods that can be used to remove oils from plant matter. It involves either submerging the plant matter in water and then turning the water into vapor or forcing steam to come into contact with the plant matter and then condensing the steam. Once the vapor is condensed, the oil can be extracted from it. This method of extraction is quick and easy, but care must be taken to control the heat and the time the plant matter is exposed to the heat because some oils can be damaged during the process.

There are a number of variations on the steam and water distillation process. Some oils require that certain compounds are added back into the oil for them to have their scent, while others require *double-distillation*, a process in which the oil is put through the distillation process twice to remove impurities.

The *expression method* is a cold-pressing method of extracting essential oils in which no heat is used during extraction. While there are a variety of expression methods in use today, they all use some sort of mechanical means to extract oil.

Chemical extraction is another method used to extract essential oil from plant matter. Solvents or hot oils are used to chemically extract the essential oil. Carbon dioxide gas has seen some use in extracting botanical oils.

The price of essential oil varies based on how difficult it is to extract the oil from the plant material.

Some essential oils will cost you less than $10 an ounce, while others might cost as much as a couple hundred an ounce. The quality of essential oils varies from manufacturer to manufacturer and can even differ from batch to batch at the same manufacturer. You're going to want to do your homework and make sure you purchase your oils in small amounts at first. Don't assume all oils are the same and buy a bunch of oil from a company you aren't familiar with. You could be setting yourself up for disappointment.

The good news is no matter how much you spend; essential oil is concentrated and will only require that you use a drop or two at a time. A small vial of essential oil will go a long way, especially if you dilute it with carrier oil before use.

Essential Oil Grades

Essential oils contain a delicate blend of naturally occurring aromatic compounds derived from seeds, stems, flowers and other plant matter. As such, the quality of the plant the oils are extracted from, along with the care taken in the extraction and cooking process, largely determines the quality of the oil.

The highest grade of essential oil available on the market today is *pure therapeutic grade oil*. This is the only type of oil you should use. Any grade of oil lower than therapeutic should be viewed as inferior and left by the wayside in favor of higher quality oils.

Pure therapeutic grade oils are made up of only the essence of the plant they are extracted from. They don't include additives or chemical substitutes added in after the extraction process to enhance the smell of the product. With pure therapeutic grade oils you get just the oil and nothing else.

There are problems associated with seeking out pure therapeutic grade oils that you need to be aware of.

As of the writing of this book, there is no government standard as to what qualifies an essential oil as therapeutic grade. The quality can vary greatly from company to company. Even when only the oils of the plant are used, the quality of the oil can be affected by extraneous factors like when the plant was harvested and how long it was left to sit around before the oil was extracted.

Another concern is contaminants in the oil. Therapeutic oils should come from organic plants that haven't been bathed in pesticides and herbicides, but there are no real controls in place to make sure this is the case. It's up to you to buy your oils from reputable companies with the proper systems of checks and balances in place to ensure you're getting high quality essential oil that works to enhance your health as opposed to being detrimental to it.

Yet another concern is the quality and type of plant being used. Different companies use different species or varieties of the plants they extract oil from. Lavender oil sold by one company isn't going to have the same qualities as lavender oil from another company. What you need to look for is oil that smells balanced and clean and absorbs quickly into the skin without leaving you feeling oily or greasy. A pure essential oil will absorb into the skin immediately upon coming into contact with it.

Grades of oil that are lower than therapeutic grade are used to flavor food and to add scent to a number of products. These lower-grade oils and floral waters have little to no therapeutic qualities left in them and should be avoided when you want to use an oil to help treat an ailment.

The Chemistry of Essential Oils

Don't worry. I'm not going to get too technical here. If you hated chemistry in high school and shudder at the thought of discussing the various natural chemical components found in essential oils, you can skip this chapter completely. It's not essential to understanding essential oils, but it will give you a better idea of what you're putting into your body and what it will do once it's in there.

The molecules found in essential oils are primarily made of carbon, hydrogen, oxygen, nitrogen and sulfur. These atoms are the building blocks of the essential oils and are what they are made of at a molecular level. The carbon atoms link together to form chains, and the other atoms stick to the chain at various points to form the oils. The chemistry of essential oils is extremely complex and this only touches the surface of their chemical composure.

Essential oils contain a number of natural chemical compounds that benefit the body in a variety of ways. Each oil is composed of its own individual blend of these compounds. No two oils are the same. This is the reason we're able to use blends of different oils to take a variety of actions in the human body.

Let's take a closer look at some of the compounds found in various essential oils.

Monoterpenes

Monoterpenes are composed of a complex combination of hydrogen and oxygen molecules that combine to form a unique compound. These helpful alcohol compounds are made up of two isoprene units and are easily oxidized. They are largely responsible for the taste and the smell of many plants.

Just to give you an idea of how complex they are; here's the structural formula for eucalyptol, which is a monoterpene found in eucalyptus oil:

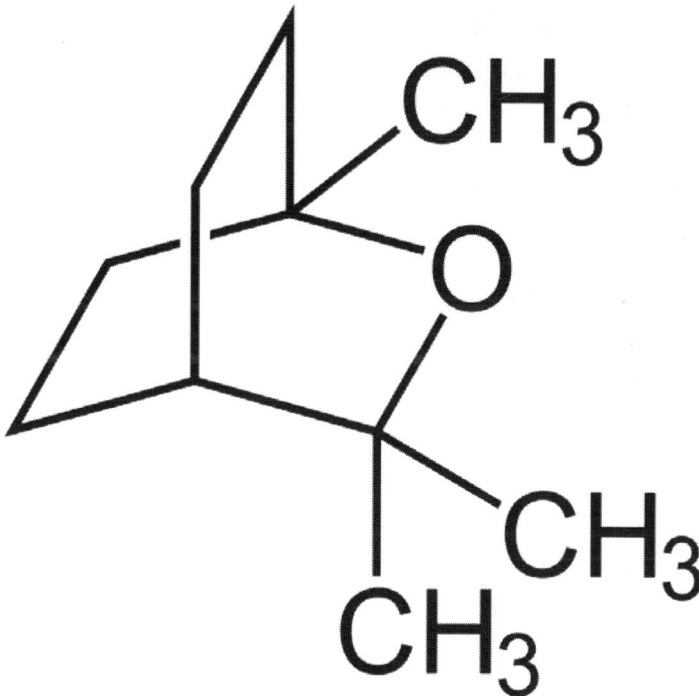

Don't worry; you don't need to memorize this structural formula. This is the one and only formula I'm going to include in the book. I just want to give you an idea of how complex a single essential oil molecule is.

Over two thousand different monoterpenes have been identified to date. Monoterpenes are said to be the life blood of many plants, and you'd be hard-pressed to find an essential oil that doesn't have any.

The following essential oils have high levels of monoterpenes:

- Angelica.
- Bay.
- Camphor.
- Caraway seed.
- Citronella.
- Citrus.
- Conifer.
- Dill.
- Eucalyptus.
- Frankincense.
- Galbanum.
- Geranium.
- Ginger.
- Hyssop.
- Juniper.
- Lemongrass.
- Myrtle.
- Neroli.
- Peppermint.
- Rose of Sharon.
- Rosewood.

- Thyme.
- Verbena.

Monoterpenes are believed to have a number of healing properties, not the least of which is to reprogram bad information in cellular DNA structure. This rewriting of bad DNA code may prevent the formation of cancerous cells. Monoterpenes are antiviral, antifungal and antiseptic by nature and are uplifting and invigorating. They prevent the build-up of toxins in the body and help remove them from the kidneys and liver.

Essential oils that are high in monoterpenes have been shown in some studies to help ease the effects of some respiratory illnesses by thinning out mucus. Taking essential oils orally has proven effective in helping acute bronchitis, chronic bronchitis and may even help alleviate some problems associated with the common cold.

It's important to note that the benefits of monoterpenes listed in this section are generalizations of monoterpene compounds in general. All monoterpene compounds are different and thus function differently in the human body.

Essential oils with high levels of monoterpenes begin to react when exposed to the air or to heat. Because they're easily oxidized, they won't last long unless properly stored in a cool, dark place.

Sesquiterpenes

Sesquiterpenes are similar to monoterpenes, except they have three isoprene units. There are more than 10,000 sesquiterpene compounds known to man.

Sesquiterpenes are thought to fight cancer by erasing or deprogramming miswritten code at the cellular level. They also deliver oxygen to cells, which creates an environment in which cancer has difficulty growing. Sesquiterpenes are anti-inflammatory, antiseptic and stimulate the immune system. They're able to pass into brain tissue from the blood and can help provide more oxygen to the brain.

The following essential oils have high levels of sesquiterpenes:

- Black Pepper.
- Blue Cypress.
- Cedarwood.
- Chamomile.
- Frankincense.
- Galbanum.
- Ginger.
- Myrhh.
- Onycha.
- Patchouli.
- Rose.
- Sandalwood.
- Spikenard.
- Vetiver.

Sesquiterpenes are less volatile than monoterpenes and don't oxidize as rapidly when exposed to air and heat.

Diterpenes

Diterpenes have four isoprene units and are less common that monoterpenes and sesquiterpenes. They are one of the biggest and heaviest molecules found in essentials oils that are created through distillation because the heavier triterpenes don't make it through distillation.

Diterpenes are found in the following essential oils:

- Cypress.
- Clary sage.
- Marijuana.
- White camphor.

These heavy compounds provide aromatic and therapeutic benefits to the oils that contain them. They have expectorant qualities and are antifungal and antimicrobial by nature.

Alcohols

Alcohols are a main building block of most essential oils. The two most common forms of alcohol found in essential oils are derivatives of monoterpenes or sesquiterpenes and are created when a carbon atom bonds to an oxygen and hydrogen molecule.

Monoterpene Alcohols

Monoterpene alcohols are abundant in essential oils. They typically don't cause irritation when applied topically.

Monoterpene alcohols can have the following beneficial qualities:

- Antibacterial.
- Antifungal.
- Antiseptic.
- Antispasmodic.
- Antiviral.
- Antimicrobial.
- May be cancer preventative.
- Diuretic.
- Sedative.

Monoterpene alcohols are abundant in the following oils:

- Citronella (contains citronellol and geraniol).
- Coriander (contains linalool).
- Eucalyptus (contains citronellol).
- Geranium (contains citronellol and geraniol).
- Jasmine (contains linalool).
- Lavender (contains linalool).

- Lemon (contains citronellol and geraniol).
- Melissa (contains citronellol).
- Palmarosa (contains geraniol).
- Rose (contains citronellol, geraniol and linalool).
- Rosewood (contains linalool).

Sesquiterpene Alcohols

Sesquiterpene alcohols aren't common in essential oils, but there are a few oils that contain them.

Sesquiterpene alcohols have the following beneficial qualities:

- Antibacterial.
- Anti-inflammatory.
- Decongestant.
- Hypoallergenic.
- Organ and gland stimulation.
- Protection against ulcers.

The following oils have elevated levels of sesquiterpene alcohols:

- German chamomile (contains bisabolol).
- Roman chamomile (contains farnesol).
- Rose (contains farnesol).
- Sandalwood (contains a-santalol).
- Ylang Ylang (contains farnesol).

Cedarwood, carrot seed and spikenard all also have specific sesquiterpene alcohols that interact with the body in a number of specific ways.

Esters

Esters are the result of *esterification*, which is a reaction between alcohol and an acid (usually acetic acid). Esters are found in a wide array of essential oils and tend to be fragrant in nature. Esters are normally well-tolerated and non-toxic and the mild oils they're abundant in can be used often. Most essential oils contain at least trace amounts of esters.

Ester compounds have the following effects on the human body:

- Antifungal.
- Anti-inflammatory.
- Antispasmodic.
- Calming.
- Easing tension.
- Muscle relaxation.
- Relaxation of the central nervous system.
- Restorative.

Oils known to be high in esters include the following:

- Bergamot.
- Birch.
- Cardamom.
- Clary sage.
- Clove.
- Cyprus.
- Jasmine.
- Lavender.
- Lemongrass.

- Orange.
- Petitgrain.
- Roman chamomile.
- Spruce.
- Sweet marjoram.
- Valerian.
- Wintergreen.
- Ylang ylang.

Aldehydes

Aldehydes are interesting in that they're irritants when applied to the skin, but have a sedative effect when they're taken into the body via inhalation.

They are often found in highly sought-after fragrances and are the driving factor behind many of the smells we're most familiar with. Both cinnamon and vanilla get their easily identifiable scents from aldehydes.

Aldehydes have the following benefits:

- Anti-inflammatory.
- Antiviral.
- Aphrodisiac.
- Calming.
- Fever reduction.
- Lower blood pressure.
- Relaxing.
- Stress relief.

The following common essential oils contain aldehydes:

- Anise (contains anisaldehyde).
- Cassia (contains cinnamaldehyde).
- Cinnamon bark (contains cinnamaldehyde).
- Citronella (contains citronellal).
- Cumin (contains cuminal).
- Lavender (contains furfural).
- Lemongrass (contains citral).
- Peppermint (contains phellandral).
- Vanilla (contains vanillin aldehyde).

While most essential oils that contain aldehydes have an aroma that's pleasant to the nose, valerian is the exception to the rule. It has a strong odor that most people find unpleasant. Don't throw out your valerian oil just yet. It's a strong sedative and can be used to help with sleeplessness if you can tolerate the smell.

Ethers

Ethers are stronger than esters and are a rarity in the most popular essential oils. In fact, they can be toxic in higher amounts and are generally avoided by those practicing aromatherapy.

The following oils contain elevated levels of ether oils and are considered to be harmful:

- Boldo.
- Calamus.
- Parsley seed.
- Sassafras.

Some ethers are suspected carcinogens when applied in concentrated amounts. Essential oils that are high in harmful ethers should be avoided unless they're being used for specific reasons and are used under the supervision of a professional. Even then, there are enough other essential oils that don't contain harmful ethers that can be used that the potential gains rarely outweigh the risks.

Not all ethers are bad news. There are some oils that contain ethers that are beneficial to the body in small amounts. These oils include anise seed, fennel, tarragon and nutmeg oil.

Ketones

You may have heard of ketones. Raspberry ketones are gaining in popularity in the fitness world. *Ketones* are formed when oxygen and carbon bond together and are similar in form to aldehydes. They have a strong fragrance when present in large amounts and can be responsible for some of the more intricate scents and flavors found in essential oils.

Ketones are thought to provide the following health benefits:

- Aids with digestion.
- Analgesic.
- Anticoagulant.
- Calming.
- Cell regeneration.
- Cold, flu and cough recovery.
- Immune system stimulation.
- Relaxation.
- Sedative.
- Tissue regeneration.
- Upper respiratory health.

The following essential oils contain ketones:

- Camphor (contains camphor).
- Caraway (contains carvone).
- Cedar bard and cedar leaf (contain thujone).
- Dill (contains carvone).
- Eucalyptus (contains piperitone).
- Fennel (contains fenchone).

- Jasmine (contains jasmine).
- Marigold (contains tagetone).
- Myrrh (contains pentanone).
- Peppermint (contains pulegone).
- Roman chamomile (contains pinocarvone).
- Rosemary (contains camphor).
- Sage (contains thyone).
- Spearmint (contains carvone).
- Vetiver (contains khusimone).

Laboratory testing on animals have shown ketones to be toxic in large dosages. They're generally considered to be safe when inhaled in small amounts.

The most toxic ketone compound found in a common essential oil is thujone, which is found in wormwood and sage oils. Thujone is a known convulsant and should be avoided by those with epilepsy as it may play a role in setting off further seizures. There are professional aromatherapists who use thujone, but this should only be done under the supervision of a professional. The stakes are too high to play around with this powerful ketone. As an interesting aside, thujone is used in absinthe, which is an alcoholic beverage that was banned for many years in the United States.

Phenols

Phenols are oxygenated compounds that contribute to the smell of the essential oils that contain them. They're powerful compounds that force the liver to work overtime, so they should only be used in small dosages and for short periods of time. They are highly caustic and can cause skin and mucous membrane irritation, so use with caution.

Phenols have the following health benefits:

- Antibacterial.
- Antimicrobial.
- Antioxidant.
- Antiseptic.
- Antispasmodic.
- May be cancer preventative.
- Oxygenating.
- Stimulant.

The following essential oils contain phenols:

- Allspice (contains eugenol).
- Basil (contains eugenol).
- Bay (contains eugenol).
- Black pepper (contains eugenol).
- Clove (contains eugenol).
- Cinnamon (contains eugenol).
- Nutmeg (contains eugenol).
- Oregano (contains thymol).
- Savory (contains carvacol).
- Thyme (contains thymol).

When oils with phenols are used, they need to be highly diluted. Never inhale, ingest or apply to your skin a full-strength oil containing phenols. They're too strong to be applied full-strength.

Oxides

Oxides form when one of the other compounds we've discussed thus far *oxidizes*. When a compound oxidizes, an oxygen atom attaches itself between two carbon atoms. Oxides have expectorant qualities and they work to thin out mucous in the respiratory system.

Eucalyptol, found in eucalyptus oil, rosemary, cinnamon, melissa and basil; is one of the most beneficial oxides found in essential oils. In addition to the expectorant qualities mentioned above, it also has antiseptic and stimulating effects on the immune system. Eucalyptol is also known as cineol.

The following essential oils are high in oxides:

- Basil (contains cineol).
- Black Peppermint (contains cineol).
- Blue mallee (contains cineol).
- Cajuput (contains cineol).
- Cardamom (contains cineol).
- Cinnamon (contains cineol).
- Clove (contains humulene oxide).
- Cypress (contains manool oxide).
- Eucalyptus (contains cineol).
- German chamomile (contains bisabolone oxide).
- Hyssop (contains linalool oxide).
- Melissa (contains cineol).
- Myrtle (contains cineol).
- Peppermint (contains piperitone oxide).
- Rose (contains rose oxide).
- Rosemary (contains cineol).

- Sage (contains cineol).
- Tea tree (contains cineol).
- Thyme (contains cineol).

Use of Essential Oils

Essential oils can be used on their own to help a person's emotional and physical well-being or they can be combined into powerful blends of oils designed for maximum benefit. What you use and how you use it is going to be a largely personal choice that should be made under the supervision of an expert in the world of holistic medicine.

There are a number of ways essential oils can be applied to the human body. The best way to apply an essential oil is largely a personal choice, and one that should be made under expert guidance.

Let's take a broad look at the various applications people are using today. Keep in mind that every application isn't suitable for every essential oil. Some oils can cause health issues when applied topically, ingested or inhaled. Doing your research beforehand will allow you to choose the proper method of application for the oil or oil blend you wish to use.

Topical Application

Pure essential oils can be applied topically, where they'll almost instantly be absorbed into the skin and transmitted throughout the body via the bloodstream.

There is a lot of literature out there that states various essential oils that are weaker in nature can be used *neat*, which means applying a few drops directly to the skin. I don't recommend this practice because some people can have severe reactions to a single drop of essential oil. Sometimes the reaction to the oil can be permanent. Your body will remember the harsh oil coming in contact with it and applying the oil later on down the road, even in diluted form, will cause an adverse reaction.

Even if your body is tolerant of using an oil neat, any more than a couple drops and you run the risk of irritation. The surrounding tissue and blood vessels may react adversely and swell up, start burning or start to itch. If this occurs, try applying carrier oil to the skin in the affected area. If irritation continues, consult with a medical professional as to your next course of action.

There are far too many ways you can apply oil in a diluted form to risk applying it neat. If you do want to use your oils undiluted, do so under the supervision of a professional aromatherapist.

Essential oils are popular with massage therapists, who use a blend of essential oils and carrier oils to create a massage oil that maximizes health benefits. Carrier oils are covered in detail later on in the book.

If you want to use multiple oils in one sitting, you may be better off buying a premixed blend of oils if you don't know what you're doing. You could also use one of the recipes found in the later chapters of this book. Haphazardly mixing essential oils and carrier oil may cause adverse reactions between certain oils which in turn may react in a different manner than what you'd expect when they're applied.

If you aren't sure whether the oils you want to apply will blend properly, you can apply them to your skin in layers instead of mixing them and applying them all at once. Apply one essential oil at a time and let it absorb completely before layering the next oil on top of it.

Hot compresses full of essential oils can be applied directly to the skin. Fill your sink full of hot water and add a few drops of some of your favorite essential oils. The oils are lighter than water and will float on top. Stir the water up, so the oils mix, and then lay a towel across the top of the water. The towel will suck the oils up as they rise to the top. Wring it out so it's damp as opposed to dripping wet and apply it to your body. Fix the compress in place and leave it for up to an hour.

Another less direct way of applying essential oils topically is to add a few drops of your favorite oils to the tub while it's filling up. This will distribute the oil evenly across your body. The oil will rise to the top of the water and will disperse itself across your skin as you stand up to get out of the tub. You'd think that since you're applying it across your whole body, more oil would be better. That isn't the case. You should only add 5 to 8 drops of oil to the tub. Any more than that and you might not be able to tolerate it.

You can also add a few drops to your favorite bath or skin care products. Adding essential oil to a shower gel or a lotion and mixing it in allows you to spread it across a larger area of your body than you would be able to if you just used the oil. It also allows you to use the stronger oils that aren't able to be applied directly.

While it isn't recommended that you use essential oils directly on your skin, I'm well-aware there are people out there who do. It stands to reason some of those people are going to read this book.

If you do decide to use one of the weaker oils like lavender oil directly on your skin, you need to be aware that any essential oil can cause an allergic reaction. The reaction can range anywhere from mild to severe and you won't know whether you're allergic to an oil until you've applied it.

The Oil Allergy Test

When you use an oil for the first time, don't use it full-strength. Dilute it with a carrier oil and apply it to a small patch of skin on an inconspicuous and hidden area of your body. Apply the oil and cover it with a bandage. Leave the bandage on for 24 hours. Remove it and check for signs of irritation.

If irritation occurs before the 24-hour mark, remove the bandage and wash your skin. If the reaction is severe, contact your local poison control center and seek immediate medical attention.

After applying heavily diluted oil, create a mixture that contains roughly twice the amount of essential oil you plan to use in your solution. If you plan on placing three drops of oil in your carrier oil when you use it for regular use, place six drops in the same amount of carrier oil. Apply it to a small patch of skin in a hidden area and cover it with a bandage for 24 hours. Watch for an allergic reaction and wash the area immediately if a reaction occurs.

If you don't have a reaction to the second test, you can probably safely use the oil along with carrier oil for topical application.

Consumption of Essential Oils

Some essential oils can be used as a dietary supplement. This is a potentially dangerous practice and should only be done under the watchful eye of a professional aromatherapist. The stakes are too high to attempt this on your own without supervision.

There are a handful of essential oils that are generally considered safe for dietary use. A good rule of thumb is to never consume an essential oil that doesn't have a nutrition facts label on the bottle. When in doubt, contact the supplier to find out whether their brand is appropriate for consumption and proceed with caution.

Again, I can't stress enough the importance of consulting with an aromatherapy professional, as well as your physician, prior to taking any essential oil internally.

Diffusion

You can reap some of the benefits of essential oils without ever having to apply them to your skin. *Diffusion* disperses essential oil into the air in the form of vapor and spreads it throughout the room in which the diffusion process takes place. In addition to having health benefits, diffused oils eliminate odors by permanently altering the molecules that create the odor. Diffused oils are even thought to fight off mold and mildew.

Be aware that harsh oils can irritate the respiratory system when diffused.

Also be aware that any method of diffusion that uses heat can alter the health benefits of the essential oil being diffused. Never allow your oils to be exposed to a direct source of heat or an open flame. They are highly-flammable and prone to rapid combustion. Cold-air diffusion methods are preferable to heat diffusion because they allow you to get the most benefit from your essential oils.

Here are some oils you can try diffusing to see if you like them:

- Bergamot.
- Frankincense.
- Lavender.
- Lemon.
- Lemongrass.
- Lime.
- Oregano.
- Patchouli.

- Peppermint.
- Pine.
- Rosewood.
- Sandalwood.
- Spruce.
- Sweet orange.
- Thyme.
- Vanilla.

The following methods can be used to diffuse essential oils into the air:

Clay Pot Diffusion

There are a number of clay and sandstone diffusion pots on the market. You place essential oil(s) in the pots and cork them shut. The essential oil slowly travels through the porous material the pot is made of and the scent eventually makes its way into the room the pot is in.

Electric Diffusers

Electric diffusers can be either air-based or heat-based. Air-based diffusers blow air across a tray or pad that contains the essential oils. The moving air picks up the scent and disperses it into the room. Air-based diffusers use cool air.

Heat-based electric diffusers have a tray into which you place your essential oil(s). When you plug it in, it heats up and disperses the scent of the oil into the room.

Glass (or Ceramic Bowl) Diffusion

Add 10 to 15 drops of essential oil to a glass bowl and let it sit out in the open. The smell of the essential oil will eventually permeate the room. To speed up the process, carry the bowl around the room before setting it in a central location.

Hot Wax Diffusion

There are a handful of ways you can diffuse your essential oils via hot wax.

The first way is to light an unscented candle and wait for the wax on top of the candle to melt. Blow the candle out and add 3 to 6 drops of essential oil to the melted wax on the top of the candle. When you relight the candle the heat will disperse the scent of the essential oil into the room the candle is placed in.

You can create your own scented candles by melting paraffin wax cubes and stirring essential oils into them. Mix your essential oils with a carrier oil first to ensure they emulsify throughout the wax. Pour the wax/oil mixture into a candle jar; add a wick; and you have your own scented candles that use essential oils instead of harsh chemicals.

Another method of dispersing essential oils through use of hot wax is to create your own scented cubes of wax and use them in a candle warmer like the Scentsy warmers. Melt a few wax cubes in a candle warmer and add a few drops of essential oil to the melted wax. Stir it up and pour the mixture into an ice cube tray. Let the wax harden and remove the wax cubes from the tray. Whenever you want to use one, pop it into your Scentsy warmer and let the smell of the essential oil permeate the room.

Lamp Ring Diffusion

Lamp rings are shaped like a donut and have a grooved edge that runs all the way around them. Add essential oil to the grooved edge; place the lamp ring over a light bulb and the heat generated by the bulb diffuses the oil into the room. This method doesn't work with HE bulbs.

Nebulizers

Nebulizers break essential oils down into a fine mist before dispersing them into the room. Instead of dispersing the scent of the oil into the room, nebulizing an oil disperses atomized particles of the oil itself. It's widely believed that this mist is more readily absorbed into the lungs than the other methods of diffusion.

The downside is there may be oils you can't use with a nebulizer because they're too heavy and won't break down and nebulizers tend to be a bit on the noisy side.

Paper Towel Diffusion

This is one of the easiest methods of diffusion and all it requires is a paper towel and some patience. Place 4 to 5 drops of essential oil on a paper towel or napkin and walk around the room while carrying it. This method works well in smaller rooms, but isn't a good choice for larger rooms.

Reed Diffusers

A reed diffuser consists of a small jar and a bunch of sticks called reeds that are placed in the jar. When you add essential oils to the jar, they travel up the reeds and the smell diffuses into the room.

Steam Diffusion

Bring a small pot of water to a boil. Remove the pot from the heat and transfer the water to a glass bowl. Drop 5 to 10 drops of essential oil in the water and let it sit. The steam will diffuse some of the essential oil into the air.

Ultrasonic Diffusers

Ultrasonic diffusers work in a manner similar to nebulizers in that they disperse a fine mist of oil into the air. A disk in the diffuser vibrates at an ultra-fast rate until it causes the essential oils to atomize. This method doesn't generate any heat and is one of the better methods to use to disperse essential oils.

Ultrasonic diffusers tend to be a bit on the expensive side, but they've come down in price in recent years. You can find a good one for less than $100.

Use of Carrier Oils to Dilute Essential Oils

Some of the stronger essential oils may need to be diluted with carrier oil. *Carrier oil* is inert oil that is used to knock down the strength of the essential oil. The proper dilution depends on the type of oil you're diluting.

They normally have a pleasant, mild scent, but can go rancid over time. If you open a container of carrier oil and it has a rank odor, your carrier oil may have gone bad.

You can use a single carrier oil to dilute your essential oils or you can create a blend. A blend of carrier oils allows you to take advantage of the health benefits associated with multiple carrier oils at the same time.

Be aware that if you're allergic to the item the oil is derived from, you're probably going to have an allergic reaction to the oil. Those with allergies to something like nuts need to take special care not just to avoid products derived from nuts, but to also avoid products made in the same area as products with nuts. Trace amounts of nut-based products can make their way into other products made in the same factory, especially if they're produced using the same machinery.

Linoleic and Oleic Fatty Acids in Carrier Oils

Carrier oils are pressed from the fatty portion of plants and tend to be high in oleic and linoleic fatty acids.

Oleic acids are omega-9 fatty acids and are widely considered to be one of the best fats to consume as part of a healthy diet. They have been shown to lower the level of bad cholesterol in the blood and help the body produce antioxidants that eliminate free radicals.

Linoleic acids are unsaturated omega-6 fatty acids that are part of a healthy diet. The body needs linoleic acids to function normally, but it can't synthesize them. They have to be consumed via the food we eat in order to enter the body.

As is the case with most things in life, you can have too much of a good thing. While using carrier oils containing linoleic and oleic fatty acids is generally considered OK for external applications like massage and aromatherapy, you need to consult with your physician before taking them orally. While these fatty acids are considered good fats, they're still fats and you need to take care if you plan on using them to supplement your diet. Most normal diets get more than enough of these fatty acids.

Fatty acids work well when applied externally because they're able to penetrate deeply into the skin. They add moisture and help heal dry and damaged skin from the inside out.

Important Safety Note about Consumption of Carrier Oils

Some of the carrier oils discussed in the rest of the chapter are labeled as being safe for consumption. It's important to note that carrier oils are vegetable oils and are used for many purposed, one of which is cooking.

Carrier oils that are labeled as safe for consumption are generally considered safe for the average person. You may have allergies that make consumption of some carrier oils unsafe. You might also have other health concerns that preclude you from being able to safely consume carrier oil as part of your diet or as a supplement to your diet.

It's of extreme importance that you realize carrier oils are not the same thing as essential oils. Once you add essential oils to a carrier oil, you change its chemical composition. Carrier oils that have been mixed with essential oils should not be consumed, even if the carrier oil is labeled as edible.

Consult with your physician before adding carrier oils to your diet.

Aloe Vera Oil

Shelf Life

Varies depending on what oil the Aloe Vera is blended with.

Aroma

Nutty.

Viscosity

Varies depending on what oil the Aloe Vera is blending with.

Benefits

Aloe Vera oil has the following benefits:

- Anti-inflammatory.
- Eases itching.
- Heals minor burns and sunburns.
- Heals skin.
- Hypoallergenic.
- Improves circulation.
- Moisturizes skin.
- Nourishes skin.
- Reduces inflammation.
- Rejuvenates skin.

Uses

Aloe Vera oil works well when applied on its own. It works even better when used as carrier oil with essential oils added to it. It can be used for massage therapy and aromatherapy.

Notes

There are only a few companies that sell Aloe Vera on its own and it's expensive to buy. Most companies that sell Aloe Vera oils are selling Aloe Vera mixed with another carrier oil. This is fine to buy and use, as pure Aloe Vera liquid is water-based and has to be mixed with an oil to get it to blend with essential oils.

Apricot Kernel Oil

Shelf Life

6 months to 1 year if stored in a cool, dark place.

Aroma

Light, slightly nutty scent that's pleasant, but not overpowering. When mixed with essential oils the scent is all but undetectable.

Viscosity

Slightly oily, but absorbs quickly and doesn't leave a residue.

Benefits

Apricot kernel oil has the following benefits:

- Anti-inflammatory.
- Antioxidant.
- High in linoleic and oleic fatty acids.
- High in vitamins A, C and E.
- Moisturizes skin.
- Nourishes skin.
- Pain relief.
- Reduces stress.
- Relieves dry, itchy skin.

Uses

Apricot kernel oil blends well with most essential oils and can be used for aromatherapy and massage therapy. It can be consumed if the oil is labeled as being edible.

Notes

Apricot kernel oil is cold-pressed from the seeds of apricots. It's a bit on the oily side, so it isn't a great choice if you're looking for something that's going to absorb right in. If, on the other hand, you're looking for a good massage oil, apricot kernel oil will probably fit the bill.

If you plan on ingesting apricot kernel oil make sure you buy unadulterated oil that's hasn't had stabilizing agents added to it. When in doubt, check with the manufacturer to see if the oil they sell is fit for consumption.

Avocado Oil

Shelf Life

6 months to 1 year if stored in a cool, dark place.

Aroma

Little to no scent.

Viscosity

Thick. Will leave skin feeling waxy if used in large amounts.

Benefits

Avocado oil has the following benefits:

- Emollient.
- High in vitamins A, B1, B2, D and E.
- Moisturizes skin.
- Nourishes skin.
- Regenerates skin.
- Relieves dry, itchy skin.
- Softens skin.

Uses

Add a small amount of avocado oil to skin and hair care products and soaps to up the nutrients. It can be added to other carrier oils and used in massage therapy.

Notes

Avocado oil penetrates deeply into the skin, leaving it feeling soft and supple.

Borage Seed Oil

Shelf Life

Up to 6 months if stored in a cool, dark place.

Aroma

Slightly sweet.

Viscosity

Thin, but leaves skin feeling oily.

Benefits

Borage seed oil has the following benefits:

- Anti-inflammatory.
- High in linoleic and oleic fatty acids.
- Moisturizes skin.
- Nourishes skin.
- Pain relief.
- Relieves dry, itchy skin.

Uses

Can be applied topically or used in aromatherapy treatments. It can also be consumed if labeled as edible, but can cause gastrointestinal problems if consumed in large amounts.

Notes

Borage seed oil is a highly sought after oil and demands a premium. The good news is a little bit goes a long way. You can blend it with other carrier oils to give them a nutritional boost.

Camellia Seed Oil

Shelf Life

Up to 2 years if stored in a cool, dark place.

Aroma

Light, slightly medicinal.

Viscosity

Somewhat oily.

Benefits

Camellia seed oil has the following benefits:

- Antioxidant.
- Emollient.
- Heartburn relief.
- High in linoleic and oleic fatty acids.
- Moisturizes skin.
- Promotes healing of damaged skin.
- Rejuvenates skin.
- Softens wrinkles.
- Strengthens nails.
- Ulcer relief.

Uses

Aromatherapy, skin and hair care products, topical application.

Notes

Camellia seed oil is also known as tea oil because it's pressed from the camellia flowers found on the same trees that grow black and green tea leaves. Don't confuse camellia seed oil with tea tree oil. Camellia seed oil is a carrier oil, while tea tree oil is a powerful essential oil.

Coconut Oil

Shelf Life

Up to 1 year if stored in a cool, dark place.

Aroma

Smells like coconuts. Cold-pressed coconut oil has almost no smell at all. Extra virgin coconut oil has a strong coconut scent.

Viscosity

Coconut oil is a solid at room temperature. When you gently warm it up, it becomes liquid. Bringing the temperature of the oil slightly above 76°F will do the trick. You can do this by placing the container in a bowl of warm water. Coconut oil melts into your skin and leaves no residue.

Benefits

Coconut oil has the following benefits:

- Calming.
- Hair care.
- May improve insulin use.
- May lower cholesterol.
- Moisturizes skin.
- Protects skin from the elements.
- Repairs damaged tissue.
- Strengthens immune system.
- Stress relief.

Uses

Aromatherapy, topical application, product creation. It can be consumed if labeled as edible.

Notes

Avoid applying coconut oil directly to the skin in sensitive areas like the face. It can cause irritation and allergic reactions.

Cranberry Seed Oil

Shelf Life

1 to 2 years if stored in a cool, dark place.

Aroma

Fruity. Tangy. Slightly pungent.

Viscosity

Thin to medium. Easily penetrates the skin. Non-greasy.

Benefits

Cranberry seed oil has the following benefits:

- Anti-inflammatory.
- Enhances cognitive function.
- High in fatty acids and vitamins A and E.
- May block UV rays (more testing is needed).
- Moisturizes skin.
- Nourishes skin.
- Relieves dry, itchy skin.
- Strong antioxidant.

Uses

Aromatherapy, topical application, product creation. Can be consumed if labeled as edible.

Notes

Cranberry seed oil is a relative newcomer to the world of carrier oils, but it brings a lot to the table. It's packed with a unique blend of nutrients that the other carrier oils don't have.

Evening Primrose Oil

Shelf Life

6 months if stored in a cool, dark place.

Aroma

Light flowery scent.

Viscosity

Somewhat oily. Leaves a light residue.

Benefits

Evening primrose oil has the following benefits:

- High in linoleic fatty acids.
- Moisturizes skin.
- Nourishes skin.
- Relieves dry, itchy skin.

Uses

Aromatherapy, topical application, product creation. Can be consumed if labeled as edible.

Notes

Evening primrose oil is expensive, but you only need to add a small amount to your carrier oil blend. Keep the amount of evening primrose oil you add to your carrier blend to between 5% and 10% to get the most bang for your buck.

Grapeseed Oil

Shelf Life

Up to 1 year if stored in a cool, dark place.

Aroma

No detectable odor.

Viscosity

Extremely light.

Benefits

Evening primrose oil has the following benefits:

- Astringent. Useful for acne and rosacea.
- High in linoleic fatty acids.
- Moisturizes skin.
- Nourishes skin.
- Regenerates skin.
- Rich in vitamins.
- Tightens skin.

Uses

Aromatherapy, topical application, product creation. Can be consumed if labeled as edible.

Notes

Grapeseed oil is a great base oil for many applications. It penetrates well and doesn't leave a residue.

Hazelnut Oil

Shelf Life

Has a long shelf life. Will last up to 2 years if stored in a cool, dark place.

Aroma

Slightly nutty.

Viscosity

Light. Little to no residue.

Benefits

Hazelnut oil has the following benefits:

- Astringent. Useful for acne and rosacea.
- High in oleic fatty acids.
- May help ease respiratory problems.
- Moisturizes skin.
- Nourishes skin.
- Regenerates skin.
- Strengthens capillaries.
- Tightens skin.

Uses

Aromatherapy, topical application, product creation. Can be consumed if labeled as edible.

Notes

Hazelnut oil is a good oil to use if you have naturally oily skin. It absorbs readily into the skin, leaving little to no residue.

Hemp Seed Oil

Shelf Life

Up to a year if stored in a cool, dark place.

Aroma

Slightly nutty.

Viscosity

Light. Leaves a slight residue.

Benefits

Hemp seed oil has the following benefits:

- Anti-inflammatory.
- Contains vitamin D and E.
- Heals damaged skin.
- High in oleic and linoleic fatty acids.
- May help ease respiratory problems.
- Moisturizes skin.
- PMS stress relief.
- Stress relief.
- Treat eczema.

Uses

Aromatherapy, topical application, product creation. Not normally consumed.

Notes

While hemp seed oil is made from hemp plants, it's important to note that the oil derived from these plants does not contain THC, which is the active ingredient in marijuana. You will not get high if you use hemp seed oil and it won't cause you to fail a drug test.

Jojoba Oil

Shelf Life

Lasts a lifetime if properly stored in a cool, dark place. Jojoba oil can be blended with other oils to extend their shelf life.

Aroma

Pleasant aroma. It's one of the stronger carrier oil aromas, but isn't off-putting. Once you've smelled it once, it's easily recognizable.

Viscosity

Medium. Jojoba oil is called an oil, but it's actually a wax. It still absorbs easily into the skin and is similar in viscosity to the oils secreted naturally by the skin.

Benefits

Jojoba oil has the following benefits:

- Acne control.
- Anti-inflammatory.
- Anti-inflammatory.
- Antioxidant.
- Cleanses skin.
- Dissolves excess sebum.
- Emollient.
- High in vitamin E.
- Moisturizes skin.

Uses

Aromatherapy, topical application, product creation. Can be consumed if labeled as edible.

Notes

Jojoba oil is a deep orange color and can interfere with some cosmetic applications. A clear version of jojoba oil is available if the bright color is a concern. It is known to clog pores when used in large amounts, so it's best to blend a small amount with other carrier oils.

Macadamia Nut Oil

Shelf Life

Up to a year if stored in a cool, dark place.

Aroma

Sweet and nutty. Has a stronger scent than most other carrier oils.

Viscosity

Medium to thick. Leaves an oily residue (or protective coating, depending on how you look at it).

Benefits

Macadamia nut oil has the following benefits:

- Anti-inflammatory.
- Contains palmitoleic acid, which is found in the natural oils of young people's skin.
- Emollient.
- Heals sunburn.
- High in oleic fatty acids.
- Moisturizes the skin.
- Promotes healing of damaged tissue and skin.
- Tones and softens skin.

Uses

Aromatherapy, topical application, product creation. Can be consumed if labeled as edible.

Notes

Macadamia nut oil should be used in small amounts as part of a carrier oil blend. The smell is too strong to be used in standalone applications.

Olive Oil

Shelf Life

Up to 2 years if stored in a cool, dark place.

Aroma

Faint scent of olives.

Viscosity

Heavy. Leaves an oily residue.

Benefits

Olive oil has the following benefits:

- High in oleic fatty acids.
- Regenerates skin cells.
- Anti-inflammatory.

Uses

Aromatherapy, topical application, product creation. Use extra virgin olive cooking oil for cooking instead.

Notes

Olive oil isn't ideal for use as a carrier oil because of its viscosity and the residue it leaves behind. If you want to use olive oil, your best bet is to add it to a carrier oil blend and only use a small amount.

Peanut Oil

Shelf Life

Up to a year if stored in a cool, dark place.

Aroma

Nutty.

Viscosity

Thick. Leaves a thick oily residue.

Benefits

Peanut oil has the following benefits:

- High in linoleic and oleic fatty acids.
- May help those with arthritis.

Uses

Peanut oil is too thick and greasy for most applications. It can be added to a massage carrier oil blend.

Notes

Avoid this oil if you have a peanut allergy as it will cause a reaction.

Rose Hip Oil

Shelf Life

Up to a year if stored in a cool, dark place.

Aroma

Earthy. Doesn't smell anything like roses.

Viscosity

Thin. Leaves a light residue.

Benefits

Rose hip oil has the following benefits:

- Helps ease the effects of a number of skin conditions.
- High in linoleic and alpha linoleic fatty acids.
- May help those with arthritis.
- Treats burns.
- Treats stretch marks.

Uses

Rose hip oil is too thick and greasy for most applications. It can be added to a massage carrier oil blend.

Notes

May aggravate acne or rosacea if used in large amounts. Blend small amounts with other oils for best results.

Sweet Almond Oil

Shelf Life

1 year if stored in a cool, dark place.

Aroma

Light, slightly nutty scent. When mixed with essential oils the scent is all but undetectable.

Viscosity

Somewhat oily. Leaves a slight residue.

Benefits

Sweet almond oil has the following benefits:

- Anti-inflammatory.
- Cold and cough relief.
- High in linoleic and oleic fatty acids.
- Moisturizes skin.
- Nourishes skin.
- Pain relief.
- Relieves dry, itchy skin.
- Relieves heartburn.

Uses

Aromatherapy, massage therapy

Notes

Sweet almond oil should be avoided by those with nut allergies. Those with diabetes should also avoid it because it may lower blood sugar to dangerous levels.

The Big List of Essential Oils

For those new to the world of essential oils and aromatherapy, the toughest part of getting started is deciding exactly what essential oils you want to buy. Unless you have an unlimited budget, you're going to need to choose the oils that are going to work best for you and your unique situation.

The following list covers many of the most popular (and some not-so-popular) essential oils available on the open market today.

Keep in mind that the price listed are as of the writing date of this book. Essential oil prices can change on a moment's notice and can vary widely from manufacturer to manufacture. The prices listed herein are a rough estimate of what you might have to pay to get a good quality oil. The price listed is the cost per ounce of oil. Most oils can be bought in quantities as small as 1/8 of an ounce, which should help you defray the cost of some of the more expensive oils.

You may notice that there is no shelf life listed for the essential oils on the Big List. This is because the shelf life varies widely from manufacturer to manufacturer and depends on a lot of extraneous factors. When in doubt, check with the company that you're buying the essential oil from. Pure essential oil doesn't go rancid, but may lose some of its aroma and health benefits over time.

African Bluegrass Oil

Price

$60 to $100 an ounce.

Derived From

African bluegrass.

Color

Light yellow.

Aroma

Sweet and grassy.

Blending

Blends well with:

- Citrus oils.
- Flower oils.

Therapeutic Properties

African bluegrass oil is said to have the following therapeutic properties:

- Antifungal.
- Antiviral.
- Astringent.

Notes

African bluegrass essential oil is primarily used to create products. It can also be diffused, added to bath water or it can be diluted and topically applied.

Agarwood Oil

Price

$250 to $500 an ounce

Derived From

Agar oil is found in the resin of hardwood that forms in Aquilaria agallocha and Gyrinops trees due to a fungal infection in the tree. The evergreen trees that agar oil is found in grow primarily in India.

Color

Deep brown.

Aroma

Deep, sweet and earthy. Very strong.

Blending

Blends well with:

- Jasmine.
- Rose.
- Sandalwood.
- Ylang ylang.

Therapeutic properties

Agarwood oil is said to have the following therapeutic properties:

- Enhanced sexual prowess.
- Good for skin.
- Relief of stress and anxiety.
- Spiritual enlightenment.

Notes

This rare oil is so expensive because it can take as long as a couple hundred years for the hardwood resin that the oil is derived from to form. Use it in small amounts to add an interesting scent to your essential oil blends. It's a popular choice for adding an interesting middle note to perfumes.

Aljwain Seed Oil

Price

$8 to $10 an ounce. You may have to buy it in larger amounts because it's relatively hard to find.

Derived From

The seeds of Bishop's weed.

Color

Pale yellow.

Aroma

Sharp and herbaceous.

Blending

Blends well with:

- Parsley.
- Thyme.
- Sage.

Therapeutic Properties

Aljwain oil is said to have the following therapeutic properties:

- Aids digestion.
- Antibacterial.
- Antifungal.
- Antiseptic.
- Germicidal.
- Is used to help with intestinal disorders.
- May help ease the effects of respiratory diseases.

- Wards off nausea.

Notes

Should not be used by pregnant women or on children. Can cause irritation to the skin.

Aljwain oil is primarily used in cosmetics, perfume and for aromatherapy.

Allspice

Price

$30 an ounce.

Derived From

The leaves or dried fruit of the pimenta dioica plant from Jamaica.

Color

Brown.

Aroma

Spicy. Reminiscent of cinnamon.

Blending

Blends well with:

- Citrus.
- Geranium.
- Ginger.
- Lavender.
- Orange.
- Patchouli.
- Spearmint.
- Sweet orange.
- Vanilla.
- Ylang ylang.

Therapeutic properties

Allspice oil is said to have the following therapeutic properties:

- Aids with indigestion.
- Antibacterial.
- Antiviral.
- Decongestant.
- May ease pain when applied topically.
- Muscle relaxant.

Notes

Allspice oil lends itself well to diffusion, but can be a mucous membrane irritant if you use too much. Be sure to only use a drop or two at a time. It's strong by nature and can cause a reaction when applied to the skin, so be sure to dilute it if you plan on applying it topically.

Amber Oil

Price

$50 to $100 an ounce.

Derived From

Tree resin. The quality of amber oil depends on the type of tree it's derived from.

Color

Clear or light yellow.

Aroma

Usually subtle and exotic, but can vary greatly depending on the type of tree used.

Blending

Blends well with:

- Cedarwood.
- Myrhh.
- Spruce.
- Pine.
- Clove.
- Aniseed.
- Citrus

Therapeutic Properties

Amber oil is said to have the following therapeutic properties:

- Antiseptic.
- Soothing.

- Eases respiratory ailments.
- Antiviral.
- May help with bladder issues.

Notes

True amber oil is a rare and precious oil and its price reflects the rarity.

Ambrette Seed Oil

Price

$200 an ounce

Derived From

The seeds of tropical hibiscus.

Color

Yellow. Almost clear.

Aroma

Woody and spicy. Floral undertones.

Blending

Blends well with:

- Amyris.
- Bergamot.
- Carrot seed.
- Exotic or spicy blends.
- Frankincense.
- Lavender.
- Myrhh.
- Patchouli.
- Peppermint.
- Spruce.

Therapeutic Properties

Ambrette seed oil is said to have the following therapeutic properties:

- Aphrodisiac.

- Eases aches and pains.
- Improves circulation.
- Stress relief.
- Stimulates adrenal gland.

Notes

Ambrette seed oil is a CO2 oil that lends itself well to perfumes. It has a unique scent that's tough to beat when it comes to essential oils. It's also diffused and can be used topically in a blend.

Amyris Oil

Price

$12 to $15 an ounce

Derived From

The wood of amyris trees.

Color

Light yellow.

Aroma

Earthy and balsamic.

Blending

Blends well with:

- Bergamot.
- Orange.
- Pine.

Therapeutic Properties

Amyris oil is said to have the following therapeutic properties:

- Calming.
- Balancing.
- May be anti-aging.
- Aphrodisiac.

Notes

Often called "West Indian Sandalwood," amyris essential oil can be used as a less-expensive alternative to sandalwood. It is commonly used in cosmetics, perfumes and soaps.

Angelica Root Oil

Price

$250.00 to $500.00 an ounce

Derived From

The roots of Angelica archangelica (wild celery).

Color

Light yellow.

Aroma

Deep and woody.

Blending

Blends well with:

- Bergamot.
- Cedarwood.
- Jasmine.
- Juniper berry.
- Orange.
- Rose.
- Sandalwood.
- Ylang ylang.

Therapeutic Properties

Angelica root oil is said to have the following therapeutic properties:

- Immune system stimulant.
- Relief of stress and anxiety.
- Revitalizes skin.

- Spiritual enlightenment.
- May ward off infection.

Notes

Avoid sunlight exposure to the area it's been applied to for at least 24 hours. Pregnant women and diabetics should avoid using angelica root oil.

Anise (or Aniseed) Oil

Price

$10 to $20 an ounce.

Derived From

The anise plant or the seeds of the anise plant.

Color

Light yellow.

Aroma

Smells like black licorice.

Blending

Blends well with:

- Black pepper.
- Caraway.
- Cedarwood.
- Coriander.
- Lavender.
- Mandarin.
- Rose.
- Rosewood.

Benefits

Anise oil is said to have the following health benefits:

- Aphrodisiac.
- Boosts stamina.
- Digestive aid.
- Energy.

- Headache relief.
- Mood enhancement.
- Nausea relief.
- May reduce cramping
- Respiratory relief.
- Stress relief.

Notes

Anise oil is potentially toxic and should be used under the supervision of an aromatherapy professional. As an interesting aside, anise oil can be used by fishermen and hunters to remove human scent from their hands prior to handling bait.

Armoise Oil

Price

$10 to $20 an ounce.

Derived From

White wormwood.

Color

Light yellow.

Aroma

Herbal and campherous.

Blending

Blends well with:

- Cedarwood.
- Clary sage.
- Lavender.
- Oak moss.
- Patchouli.
- Pine.
- Rosemary.
- Sage.

Therapeutic Properties

Armoise oil is said to have the following therapeutic properties:

- Aids digestive system.
- Antiseptic.
- Kills intestinal worms.

- Local anesthetic.
- Pain relief.

Notes

Armoise oil is potentially toxic if ingested. Only use it under the supervision of an aromatherapy professional.

Balsam Peru Oil

Price

$10 an ounce.

Derived From

The bark of myroxylon pereirae trees, native to South and Central America.

Color

Dark brown.

Aroma

Fresh, reminiscent of vanilla.

Blending

Blends well with:

- Most essential oils.

Therapeutic Properties

Balsam Peru oil is said to have the following therapeutic properties:

- May ease the effects of scabies.
- Helps the user focus.
- Relaxing.
- Relieves stress.

Notes

Balsam Peru oil is a popular scent that's often added to perfumes. It doesn't lend well to topical application, as it can cause an allergic reaction.

Basil Oil

Price

$25 to $40 an ounce.

Derived From

Basil.

Color

Clear to light yellow or light green.

Aroma

Spicy, with a hint of pepper.

Blending

Blends well with:

- Bergamot.
- Citrus oils.
- Eucalyptus.
- Frankincense.
- Lemon.
- Spice oils.

Therapeutic Properties

Basil oil is said to have the following therapeutic properties:

- Antibacterial.
- Antiseptic.
- Antispasmodic.
- Headache relief.
- Heals and nourishes the skin.

- Thought to help ease the effects of PMS.
- Memory improvement.
- Muscle ache relief.
- Relaxing.
- Relieves stress.
- Respiratory disorder relief.

Notes

Basil essential oil is commonly used to make perfumes and is also used in aromatherapy. It has an overpowering scent and should only be used in small amounts. It contains a substance called methyl chavicol that is thought to be carcinogenic in large amounts and may contribute to other health issues. Use basil oil sparingly and seek out high-quality oils that are low in methyl chavicol.

Basil oil should not be given to women who are pregnant or children. It's a strong oil and can irritate sensitive skin, so always test in a small area prior to application.

Bay Oil

Price

$15 to $75 an ounce, depending on the type of bay leaves it's harvested from.

Derived From

Bay leaves. There is a wide array of varieties of bay leaf that bay essential oil may be derived from.

Color

Golden.

Aroma

Varies. Tends to be strong and spicy.

Blending

Blends well with:

- Bergamot.
- Clary sage.
- Frankincense.
- Juniper.
- Patchouli.
- Ylang ylang.

Therapeutic Properties

Bay oil is said to have the following therapeutic properties:

- Anticonvulsant.
- Antifungal.
- Antiseptic.
- Bug repellant.

- Decongestant.
- May heal skin problems.
- Pain relief.
- Relaxing.
- Soothes itching.

Notes

Bay leaf oil is a popular choice for perfumes and cosmetics. It's also a popular choice for massage oils and diffusion. Always dilute with carrier oil before applying bay essential oil topically. Bay oil can irritate the mucous membranes, so use it sparingly.

Bay leaf oil and bay laurel oil are two different oils. They're commonly confused with one another because they have a similar name and similar properties.

Bay Laurel Oil

Price

$40 to $70 an ounce.

Derived From

Bay laurel leaves.

Color

Very light yellow.

Aroma

Camphor.

Blending

Blends well with:

- Bergamot.
- Eucalyptus.
- Helichrysum.
- Lavender.
- Rosemary.
- Ylang ylang.

Therapeutic Properties

Bay laurel oil is said to have the following therapeutic properties:

- Antifungal.
- Antiseptic.
- Decongestant.
- Diuretic.
- Thought to heal and protect the skin.

- May lower blood pressure.
- Promotes confidence.

Notes

Bay laurel oil is commonly used in diffusers. Avoid topical application as it can irritate the skin. This oil is as close to a complete oil as you're probably going to get, as it contains a large number of various beneficial chemical compounds.

Bay leaf oil and bay laurel oil are two different oils. They're commonly confused with one another because they have a similar name and similar properties.

Bergamot (Bitter Orange) Oil

Price

$30 an ounce.

Derived From

The peels of bitter oranges.

Color

Green.

Aroma

Sweet and tangy citrus. The scent varies dependent upon whether or not the fruit is ripe when it's picked.

Blending

Blends well with:

- Citrus oils.
- Frankincense.
- Wood oils.

Therapeutic Properties

Bergamot oil is said to have the following therapeutic properties:

- Antibacterial.
- Antidepressant.
- Antiseptic.
- Antispasmodic.
- Aphrodisiac.
- Balances skin.
- Calming.

- Elevates mood.
- Relaxing.
- Stress relief.

Notes

Bergamot essential oil is popular in perfumes and is used in aromatherapy. It's a bit strong for topical application, so only use a drop mixed with carrier oil and test in an inconspicuous area if you plan on applying it to your skin.

It contains a chemical that's known to be phototoxic, so avoid allowing the sun to contact the area where it was applied for at least 48 hours.

Birch Oil

WARNING: Birch oil contains a chemical compound (methyl salicylate) that is converted to salicylic acid in the body. *Salicylic acid* is similar to aspirin, so birch oil should not be used by those who are allergic to aspirin. If used, it needs to be used under the supervision of a doctor and should only be used for short periods of time.

Price

$15 to $20 an ounce.

Derived From

The bark of birch trees.

Color

Pale green.

Aroma

Minty and woody.

Blending

Blends well with:

- Wood oils.

Therapeutic Properties

Birch oil is said to have the following therapeutic properties:

- Analgesic.
- Anti-inflammatory.
- Astringent.
- Decongestant.

- Diuretic.
- Pain relief.
- Relaxing.
- Soothes and loosens muscles.

Notes

Birch oil is a heavy oil. It's one of the few oils that sinks when added to water. It's often used as a more refined substitute for wintergreen. Always dilute birch essential oil and only use it in small amounts.

Black Pepper Oil

Price

$25 to $30 an ounce.

Derived From

Ripe pepper fruit.

Color

Yellow.

Aroma

Spicy and earthy, with floral undertones.

Blending

Blends well with:

- Basil.
- Cedarwood.
- Lavender.
- Marjoram.
- Sandalwood.

Therapeutic Properties

Black pepper oil is said to have the following therapeutic properties:

- Aphrodisiac.
- Improves circulation.
- Loosens muscles.
- Relieves aches and pains.
- Stimulant.

Notes

The scent of black pepper essential oil is understated and can be used to add a spicy floral scent to your oil blends. It should be used in small amounts if you plan on applying it topically, as it can irritate the skin.

Cacao Absolute Oil

Price

$20 to $30 an ounce

Derived From

Cocoa beans.

Color

Brown.

Aroma

Smells like fine dark chocolate.

Blending

Blends well with:

- Cinnamon.
- Citrus.
- Patchouli.
- Peppermint.
- Vanilla.
- Wood oils.

Therapeutic Properties

Cacao oil is said to have the following therapeutic properties:

- Nourishes and moisturizes skin.
- Stress relief.

Notes

Cacao oil is a popular choice for aromatherapy and is often added to skin care products and oil blends in small amounts to give it a hint of chocolate scent.

Cade Oil

Price

$50 to $100 an ounce.

Derived From

The wood of the prickly juniper tree.

Color

Brown.

Aroma

Earthy and woody.

Blending

Blends well with:

- Clove.
- Rosemary.
- Thyme.
- Wood oils.

Therapeutic Properties

Cade oil is said to have the following therapeutic properties:

- Analgesic.
- Antimicrobial.
- Antiseptic.
- Disinfectant.
- Used for a number of skin problems.

Notes

Cade essential oil is typically used in ointments and creams. Cade oil contains carcinogenic compounds and should only be used under supervision, if at all.

Cajeput Oil

Price

$5 to $10 an ounce.

Derived From

The leaves of the cajeput tree.

Color

Light yellow, almost clear.

Aroma

Camphorous, like eucalyptus.

Blending

Blends well with:

- Cedarwood.
- Clove.
- Rosemary.
- Thyme.

Therapeutic Properties

Cajeput oil is said to have the following therapeutic properties:

- Antibacterial.
- Concentration.
- Eases effects of colds.
- Expectorant.
- Improves mood.
- Relieves muscle stiffness and pain.
- Stress relief.

Notes

Cajeput oil is commonly used in massage oils, skin care products and perfumes. It's also a good choice for those wanting to diffuse their essential oil. It may cause skin irritation, so use in small amounts and test in a small area prior to application.

Calamus Root Oil

Price

$10 to $20 an ounce.

Derived From

The root of the calamus plant.

Color

Dark yellow.

Aroma

Smells spicy. Reminiscent of cinnamon.

Blending

Blends well with:

- Bitter orange.
- Clary sage.
- Lavender.
- Patchouli.
- Rosemary.
- Spice oils.

Therapeutic Properties

Calamus root oil is said to have the following therapeutic properties:

- Antibacterial.
- Antibiotic.
- Improves circulation.
- Stimulant.

Notes

Use calamus root essential oil in small amounts, as larger dosages can leave you feeling like you're walking around in a daze. This product contains asarone, which is a potentially toxic compound. Always use under the supervision of an aromatherapy specialist.

Calendula (Marigold) Oil

Price

$35 to $45 an ounce

Derived From

Calendula flowers.

Color

Yellow or green.

Aroma

Floral and slightly citrus.

Blending

Blends well with:

- Citrus oils.
- Floral oils.
- Wood oils.

Therapeutic Properties

Calendula oil is said to have the following therapeutic properties:

- Antibacterial.
- Anti-inflammatory.
- Antioxidant.
- Antiseptic.
- Eases insect stings and bites.
- Good for dry skin.
- May aid with tissue regeneration.
- May help ward off cancer.

- Stimulant.

Notes

Calendula essential oil is typically added to oil blends or skin care products in small amounts and applied topically. It's widely considered to be nontoxic and is a good choice for people with sensitive or irritated skin.

Camphor Oil (White)

Price

$6 to $10 an ounce.

Derived From

The wood of camphor trees.

Color

Brown.

Aroma

Camphorous. Are you surprised?

Blending

Blends well with:

- Citrus oils.
- Lavender.
- Melissa.
- Spice oils.

Therapeutic Properties

White camphor oil is said to have the following therapeutic properties:

- Antidepressant.
- Decongestant.
- Used for skin problems.

Notes

WARNING: Camphor oil is a toxic oil that contains a substance that's a known carcinogen. White camphor oil is supposedly safer than camphor oil, but you'd better be sure you're getting your oil from a reputable supplier. I recommend only using white camphor oil under the supervision of an aromatherapy professional.

White camphor oil is used in tiger balms and rubs. It's also used for aromatherapy, but should only be used in small amounts for this purpose.

Cananga Oil

Price

$3 to $10 an ounce.

Derived From

The flowers of the cananga tree.

Color

Yellow.

Aroma

Woody and floral.

Blending

Blends well with:

- Cassia.
- Lavender.
- Rose.
- Rosemary.

Therapeutic Properties

Cananga oil is said to have the following therapeutic properties:

- Antidepressant.
- Antiseptic.
- Aphrodisiac.
- Helps prevent infection.
- Stimulant.

Notes

Cananga can be used as a less-expensive alternative to ylang ylang oil. Use small amounts, as it can cause moderate to severe headaches when used in larger amounts. It can cause a reaction if it's used on the skin.

Caraway Seed Oil

Price

$15 to $40 an ounce.

Derived From

Carum carvi seeds.

Color

Light yellow, almost clear.

Aroma

Warm and spicy. Strong.

Blending

Blends well with:

- Bay.
- Black Pepper.
- Chamomile.
- Cinnamon.
- Citrus oils.
- Ginger.
- Jasmine.
- Lavender.

Therapeutic Properties

Caraway seed oil is said to have the following therapeutic properties:

- Antiseptic.
- Antispasmodic.
- Astringent.

- May open breathing passages.
- Revitalizing.

Notes

Also known as meadow cumin oil, caraway oil is nontoxic and can be used for most aromatherapy applications. It can irritate the skin if used in large amounts.

Cardamom Oil

Price

$60 an ounce.

Derived From

Cardamom fruit or seeds.

Color

Clear.

Aroma

Amazing (Yes, this is the author's bias). Woody and spicy.

Blending

Blends well with:

- Most essential oils.

Therapeutic Properties

Cardamom essential oil is said to have the following therapeutic properties:

- Antispasmodic.
- Aphrodisiac.
- Cold relief.
- Energy.
- Expectorant.
- Libido.
- Stress relief.

Notes

This is one of the author's personal favorite oils because of it' interesting and unique scent. I prefer to diffuse it all by itself, but it can be added to other oils to make unique and intricate blends. It's a little pricey, but you'll get a lot of mileage from your cardamom essential oil because a little bit goes a long way.

Carrot Seed Oil

Price

$25 to $75 an ounce.

Derived From

The seeds of the carrot plant.

Color

Yellow to orange.

Aroma

Woody and sweet.

Blending

Blends well with:

- Bergamot.
- Cedarwood.
- Cinnamon.
- Citrus oils.
- Juniper.
- Lavender.

Therapeutic Properties

Carrot seed oil is said to have the following therapeutic properties:

- Improves circulation.
- Nourishes and moisturizes skin.
- Reduces effects of PMS.
- Thought to remove blemishes.
- Thought to reduce wrinkles.

- Used on skin conditions.

Notes

Carrot seed essential oil is used in skin care products. It is safe to use, but is phototoxic. You need to avoid sun exposure for at least 24 hours after applying products containing carrot seed oil. Pregnant women should steer clear of carrot seed oil.

Cassia Oil

Price

$5 to $15 an ounce.

Derived From

The evergreen cassia tree.

Color

Yellow to brown.

Aroma

Spicy and pungent.

Blending

Blends well with:

- Frankincense.
- Ginger.
- Lavender.
- Myrrh.
- Spice oils.

Therapeutic Properties

Cassia oil is said to have the following therapeutic properties:

- Antibacterial.
- Antifungal.
- Antiseptic.
- May lower blood pressure.
- Sedative.
- Stimulant.

Notes

Cassia oil is a powerful oil that can be a dermal irritant if applied topically. It can also irritate mucous membranes. It's recommended that you use this oil under the supervision of an aromatherapy professional.

Catnip Oil

Price

$50 to $100 an ounce.

Derived From

Catnip.

Color

Deep yellow.

Aroma

Minty.

Blending

Blends well with:

- Cedarwood.
- Citronella.
- Eucalyptus.
- Geranium.
- Peppermint.

Therapeutic Properties

Catnip oil is said to have the following therapeutic properties:

- Anti-inflammatory.
- Headache relief.
- Insect repellent.
- Pain relief.
- Promotes menstruation.
- Stress relief.

- Used to ease the effects of the common cold.

Notes

Avoid use during pregnancy and don't use on small children. The long-term effects of catnip essential oil as an aromatherapy treatment are unknown.

Cedarwood Oil

Price

$5 to $10 an ounce

Derived From

The wood of cedar trees. The variety of cedar tree varies from manufacturer to manufacturer.

Color

Yellow or green.

Aroma

Campherous and earthy.

Blending

Blends well with:

- Citrus oils.
- Eucalyptus.
- Juniper.
- Rose.
- Rosemary.
- Sandalwood.
- Vetivert.

Therapeutic Properties

Cedarwood oil is said to have the following therapeutic properties:

- Antidepressant.
- Antifungal.
- Antiseptic.

- Clarity of mind.
- Focus.
- Improved urine flow.
- Insect repellant.

Notes

Cedarwood is one of the more powerful essential oils for aromatherapy purposes. It clears the mind and grounds the soul, preparing you for what's to come in the near future. Be aware that cedarwood essential oil contains a high level of hydrocarbons that may damage the lungs.

Celery Seed Oil

Price

$80 to $100 an ounce.

Derived From

The seeds of celery plants.

Color

Yellow.

Aroma

Earthy.

Blending

Blends well with:

- Black pepper.
- Lavender.
- Tea tree.

Therapeutic Properties

Celery seed oil is said to have the following therapeutic properties:

- Calming.
- Diuretic.
- Menstrual health.
- Relaxing.
- Urinary health.
- Warming.

Notes

Celery seed essential oil is used in perfumes, skin care products and massage oils.

Chamomile Oil

Price

$60 to $180 an ounce.

Derived From

Chamomile plant.

Color

Blue.

Aroma

Fruity and herbaceous.

Blending

Blends well with:

- Citrus oils.
- Flower oils.
- Frankincense.
- Lavender.
- Spice oils.
- Tea tree.

Therapeutic Properties

Chamomile oil is said to have the following therapeutic properties:

- Antidepressant.
- Anti-inflammatory.
- Calming.
- Clears the mind.
- Combats insomnia.

- Relaxing.
- Sedative.
- Stress relief.

Notes

There are a ton of chamomile oils on the market. When it comes to aromatherapy, the only two you should use are German chamomile and Roman chamomile. Of the two, I'd go with Roman chamomile, as it's one of the safer and more robust oils on the market. It's widely considered safe for use with children as long as it's heavily diluted.

Roman chamomile is safe to use for most aromatherapy uses.

Cinnamon Oil

Price

$25 to $75 an ounce.

Derived From

The bark or leaves of the cinnamon tree.

Color

Light brown or green.

Aroma

Smells like cinnamon.

Blending

Blends well with:

- Bitter orange.
- Frankincense.
- Geranium.
- Lavender.
- Lemon.
- Patchouli.

Therapeutic Properties

Cinnamon oil is said to have the following therapeutic properties:

- Antibacterial.
- Antimicrobial.
- Improved blood flow.
- Sexual stimulant.

Notes

Keep away from sensitive areas of the skin, as cinnamon essential oil can be an irritant. If you plan on using it topically, heavily dilute it, test it first and make sure you can tolerate it, and then only use it in small amounts.

Because of its strong scent, cinnamon essential oil lends itself well to diffusion.

Cistus Oil

Price

$45 to $55 an ounce.

Derived From

The leaves of the cistus shrub.

Color

Green.

Aroma

Floral and herbaceous. Reminiscent of eucalyptus.

Blending

Blends well with:

- Angelica.
- Citrus oils.
- Frankincense.
- Patchouli.
- Wood oils.

Therapeutic Properties

Cistus oil is said to have the following therapeutic properties:

- Anti-inflammatory.
- Disinfectant.
- Heals and nourishes skin.
- May ease the effects of respiratory problems.
- Relaxing.
- Stress relief.

Notes

Cistus essential can be diffused or used in skin care products. It's generally considered to be non-toxic. Use it in small amounts to enhance the scent of your oil blends. More than a drop or two tends to crowd out other smells.

Citronella Oil

Price

$5 to $10 an ounce.

Derived From

Citronella grass.

Color

Light yellow, almost clear.

Aroma

Sweet and fresh.

Blending

Blends well with:

- Eucalyptus.
- Lavender.
- Lemongrass.
- Peppermint.
- Vanilla.

Therapeutic Properties

Citronella oil is said to have the following therapeutic properties:

- Antibacterial.
- Antidepressant.
- Antiseptic.
- Antispasmodic.
- Calming.
- Diuretic.

- Relaxing.
- Strong bug repellent.

Notes

Citronella is mainly used as an insect repellant, but it has a lot of other beneficial qualities. It can be diffused or added to skin care products or candles.

Clary Sage Oil

Price

$15 to $75 an ounce.

Derived From

Clary sage, an herb native to Southern Europe.

Color

Light yellow.

Aroma

Earthy and floral.

Blending

Blends well with:

- Bergamot.
- Chamomile.
- Floral oils.
- Frankincense.
- Orange.
- Sandalwood.
- Ylang ylang.

Therapeutic Properties

Clary sage oil is said to have the following therapeutic properties:

- Anticonvulsant.
- Antidepressant.
- Antiseptic.
- Antispasmodic.

- Aphrodisiac.
- Deodorant.
- PMS and menopause relief.
- Relaxing.
- Sedative.
- Stress relief.

Notes

Clary sage essential oil has slightly narcotic properties and shouldn't be used before driving or operating heavy machinery. It should also be avoided by pregnant women.

It's commonly used to add scent to a number of natural skin care products. It can be diffused or added to massage oil and applied topically.

Clove Oil

Price

$15 to $50 an ounce.

Derived From

The leaves or buds of the clove tree.

Color

Clear to light yellow.

Aroma

Spicy. Overpowering in large amounts.

Blending

Blends well with:

- Citrus oils.
- Peppermint.
- Spice oils.

Therapeutic Properties

Clove oil is said to have the following therapeutic properties:

- Analgesic.
- Antibacterial.
- Antiseptic.
- Antispasmodic.
- Disinfectant.
- Fights infection.
- Respiratory relief.
- Stimulant.

Notes

Clove essential oil is very strong. Exercise caution and dilute your clove oil heavily, especially if you're planning on applying it topically. Always test a small area first. It can be used in a diffuser, in skin care products or as part of a massage oil.

Coffee Oil

Price

$25 to $40 an ounce.

Derived From

Coffee beans.

Color

Brown.

Aroma

Strong coffee.

Blending

Use coffee essential oil as a standalone oil. The scent overpowers other oils.

Therapeutic Properties

Coffee oil is said to have the following therapeutic properties:

- Antidepressant.
- Antioxidant.
- Deodorant.
- Helps ease respiratory problems.

Notes

Diffuse coffee essential oil in a room you want to deodorize. Be careful, because it can cause irregular heartbeat in some people. Do not use if pregnant.

Coriander Oil

Price

$15 to $20 an ounce.

Derived From

The seeds of the coriander plant.

Color

Light yellow.

Aroma

Woody and campherous.

Blending

Blends well with:

- Black Pepper.
- Cinnamon.
- Citronella.
- Jasmine.
- Most spice oils.
- Petitgrain.
- Sandalwood.

Therapeutic Properties

Coriander oil is said to have the following therapeutic properties:

- Analgesic.
- Antibacterial.
- Antifungal.
- Anti-inflammatory.

- Antioxidant.
- Antispasmodic.
- Aphrodisiac.
- Cleansing.
- Happiness.
- Nervous system stimulant.
- Promotes healthy skin.
- Uplifting.

Notes

Coriander essential oil is widely considered safe when used in small dosages for aromatherapy purposes. In larger doses, it can have a sedative effect, so use with caution and keep the amount you include in your blends to a minimum.

Cubeb Oil

Price

$30 an ounce.

Derived From

The fruit of the cubeb plant.

Color

Light yellow.

Aroma

Woody and campherous.

Blending

Blends well with:

- Bergamot.
- Floral oils.
- Spice oils.
- Ylang ylang.

Therapeutic Properties

Cubeb oil is said to have the following therapeutic properties:

- Anti-inflammatory.
- Antiseptic.
- Astringent.
- Relaxing.
- Stress relief.

Notes

Cubeb essential oil may irritate the skin. Dilute heavily and test in a small area before application.

Cumin Oil

Price

$30 to $50 an ounce.

Derived From

Cumin seeds.

Color

Light yellow.

Aroma

Spicy.

Blending

Blends well with:

- Caraway.
- Chamomile.
- Coriander.
- Lavender.
- Spice oils.

Therapeutic Properties

Cumin oil is said to have the following therapeutic properties:

- Antibacterial.
- Antiseptic.
- Antispasmodic.
- Diuretic.
- Stimulant.

Notes

Cumin essential oil is phototoxic. If you apply it topically, avoid sunlight exposure for at least 24 hours. It shouldn't be used by pregnant women. Only use small amounts because it's been known to cause headaches with larger dosages.

Cypress Oil

Price

$50 to $100 an ounce.

Derived From

The branches of cypress trees.

Color

Light yellow. Almost clear.

Aroma

Woody and spicy. Hints of pine.

Blending

Blends well with:

- Citrus oils.
- Clary sage.
- Fennel.
- Jasmine.
- Lavender.
- Wood oils.

Therapeutic Properties

Cypress oil is said to have the following therapeutic properties:

- Antidepressant.
- Calming.
- Helps with respiratory conditions.
- Relaxing.
- Soothing.

- Stress relief.

Notes

Cypress essential oil works great when used for masculine products that you want to imbibe with a manly scent. It is generally considered to be non-toxic, but should be avoided by pregnant women. This oil is a favorite amongst aromatherapy practitioners and lends itself well to most uses.

Davana Oil

Price

$150 to $200 an ounce.

Derived From

Davana flowers and leaves.

Color

Green to brown.

Aroma

Fruity.

Blending

Blends well with:

- Black pepper.
- Jasmine.
- Orange.
- Patchouli.
- Rose.
- Spikenard.
- Tuberose.
- Vanilla.
- Wood oils.
- Ylang ylang.

Therapeutic Properties

Davana oil is said to have the following therapeutic properties:

- Antiseptic.

- Antiviral.
- Aphrodisiac.
- Disinfectant.
- Moisturizes the skin.

Notes

Davana oil has an interesting quality when applied topically. It interacts with the skin to create a scent that's unique to the person it was applied to. You never know exactly what you're going to get. The good news is it's almost always a pleasingly fruity scent.

Davana oil can be used for most aromatherapy purposes, but works best when diffused into the air. It may irritate skin when applied topically and should be avoided by pregnant women.

Dill Seed Oil

Price

$15 to $20 an ounce.

Derived From

Dried dill seeds.

Color

Light yellow.

Aroma

Smells like dill pickles.

Blending

Blends well with:

- Spice oils.
- Peppermint.

Therapeutic Properties

Dill seed oil is said to have the following therapeutic properties:

- Aid in healing damaged skin.
- Calming.
- Insect repellant.
- May help regulate glucose levels.
- May help with insomnia and other sleep disorders.
- Purifying.
- Relaxing.
- Relieves stress and anxiety.
- Sedative.

- Believed to stimulate milk flow in nursing mothers.

Notes

Dill seed essential oil can be used for most aromatherapy purposes.

Douglas Fir Needle Oil

Price

$20 to $30 an ounce.

Derived From

The needles of the Douglas fir tree.

Color

Light yellow. Almost clear.

Aroma

Woody and sweet.

Blending

Blends well with:

- Frankincense.
- Lavender.
- Lemon.
- Other evergreen oils.

Therapeutic Properties

Douglas fir needle oil is said to have the following therapeutic properties:

- Antidepressant.
- Anti-infectious.
- Eases aches and pains.
- May help with respiratory conditions.
- Relieves muscle aches and pains.
- Uplifting.

Notes

Douglas fir essential oil works well when diffused or when blended with other oils and applied topically. Always test in a small area first.

Elemi Oil

Price

$15 an ounce.

Derived From

Elemi tree resin.

Color

Clear.

Aroma

Woody and balsamic.

Blending

Blends well with:

- Spice oils.
- Wood oils.

Therapeutic Properties

Elemi oil is said to have the following therapeutic properties:

- Analgesic.
- Antibacterial.
- Antifungal.
- Anti-inflammatory.
- Antimicrobial.
- Antiseptic.
- Antiviral.
- Expectorant.

Notes

Elemi essential works well when diffused or applied topically. It's one of the more gentle essential oils and can usually be applied directly to the skin at full strength. Always test in an inconspicuous area first and only apply a few drops at a time.

Eucalyptus Oil

Price

$20 to $40 an ounce.

Derived From

The branches and leaves of eucalyptus trees.

Color

Light yellow or light green. Almost clear.

Aroma

Woody and campherous.

Blending

Blends well with:

- Bergamot.
- Juniper.
- Lavender.
- Lemon.
- Lemongrass.
- Rosemary.
- Thyme.
- Wood oils.

Therapeutic Properties

Eucalyptus oil is said to have the following therapeutic properties:

- Antibacterial.
- Antifungal.
- Antiseptic.

- Deodorant.
- Decongestant.
- Immune system stimulant.
- Used to ease effects of colds and the flu.

Notes

Eucalyptus essential oil is a strong oil that needs to be heavily diluted before being used for aromatherapy purposes. It should be avoided by pregnant women and those with high blood pressure, and should never be taken internally.

Erigeron Oil

Price

$15 to $150 an ounce.

Derived From

Fleabane plants.

Color

Light yellow.

Aroma

Fresh and spicy.

Blending

Blends well with:

- Cardamom.
- Cilantro.
- Citrus oils.
- Spearmint.

Therapeutic Properties

Erigeron oil is said to have the following therapeutic properties:

- Antispasmodic.
- Balancing.
- Insect repellant.
- Stimulant.

Notes

Erigeron essential oil is a relatively unknown oil only provided by a small handful of essential oil suppliers. It's primarily used for its bug repellant qualities. People swear by its ability to repel fleas.

Fennel Oil

Price

$15 to $20 an ounce.

Derived From

Fennel herb seeds.

Color

Light yellow.

Aroma

Sweet and spicy.

Blending

Blends well with:

- Anise.
- Bergamot.
- Frankincense.
- Geranium.
- Lavender.
- Rose.
- Rosemary.
- Sandalwood.
- Spice oils.

Therapeutic Properties

Fennel oil is said to have the following therapeutic properties:

- Antiseptic.
- Antispasmodic.

- Can be used to treat colic.
- Eases indigestion.
- Expectorant.
- May stop hair loss.
- Promotes healthy skin.
- Used to help with bruising.

Notes

Fennel essential oil is powerful and needs to be diluted heavily when used for aromatherapy purposes. It can cause skin irritation and contains chemicals that may promote cancer growth when used in large amounts.

Frankincense Oil

Price

$15 to $100 an ounce.

Derived From

Frankincense resin.

Color

Light yellow.

Aroma

Earthy and warm.

Blending

Blends well with:

- Basil.
- Bergamot.
- Citrus oils.
- Chamomile.
- Cinnamon.
- Geranium.
- Lavender.
- Myrrh.
- Pine.
- Sandalwood.
- Vanilla.

Therapeutic Properties

Frankincense oil is said to have the following therapeutic properties:

- Antiseptic.
- Astringent.
- Calming.
- Diuretic.
- Expectorant.
- Grounding.
- Sedative.

Notes

Along with myrrh, frankincense is probably the most well-known essential oil because of its Biblical ties. It's generally considered to be nontoxic, but should be avoided by pregnant women nonetheless.

Frankincense essential oil can be used for most aromatherapy applications.

Galanga Oil

Price

$15 to $20 an ounce.

Derived From

False ginger.

Color

Yellow.

Aroma

Clean, spicy and campherous.

Blending

Blends well with:

- Cardamom.
- Chamomile.
- Cinnamon.
- Ginger.
- Patchouli.
- Sage.

Therapeutic Properties

Galanga oil is said to have the following therapeutic properties:

- Antibacterial.
- Antispasmodic.
- Calming.
- Relieves nausea.

Notes

Galanga essential oil needs to be used with caution because it can cause hallucinations when large amounts are used. It can also interact negatively with a number of prescription and over-the-counter drugs.

Galbanum Oil

Price

$40 to $50 an ounce.

Derived From

Galbanum gum.

Color

Light yellow.

Aroma

Spicy and fresh.

Blending

Blends well with:

- Evergreen oils.
- Frankincense.
- Lavender.
- Myrrh.
- Oak moss.
- Violet.

Therapeutic Properties

Galbanum oil is said to have the following therapeutic properties:

- Anti-inflammatory.
- Antispasmodic.
- Heals skin.
- Pain relief.

Notes

Galbanum essential oil can be used for most aromatherapy purposes.

Garlic Oil

Price

$20 to $40 an ounce.

Derived From

Garlic cloves.

Color

Yellow to orange.

Aroma

Smells like garlic.

Blending

Garlic oil has a strong, pungent scent that doesn't lend well to blending.

Therapeutic Properties

Garlic oil is said to have the following therapeutic properties:

- Antibacterial.
- Anticoagulant.
- Anti-inflammatory.
- Antiseptic.
- Insect repellant.
- May lower blood pressure.
- Promotes healing.
- Rejuvenating.

Notes

Garlic essential oil has its benefits, but is difficult to use because of the strong garlic odor that makes itself known to everyone in the general area. It can be used for most aromatherapy purposes, but many people avoid it because of the difficulty of use.

Geranium Oil

Price

$70 to $100 an ounce.

Derived From

Geranium leaves.

Color

Brown.

Aroma

Floral. Similar to rose oil.

Blending

Blends well with:

- Fennel.
- Frankincense.
- Grapefruit.
- Lemon.
- Most spice oils.
- Rose.
- Rosewood.
- Ylang ylang.

Therapeutic Properties

Geranium oil is said to have the following therapeutic properties:

- Antibacterial.
- Antidepressant.
- Antifungal.

- Anti-inflammatory.
- Expectorant.
- Insect repellent.
- Promote skin healing and health.
- Stress relief.

Notes

This pleasant oil can be used for most aromatherapy applications. It's most common application is as an additive to rose oil. Geranium oil is thought to imbalance the hormones of some people, so it's recommend that you use it under professional supervision.

Ginger Oil

Price

$10 to $20 an ounce.

Derived From

Ginger root.

Color

Yellow.

Aroma

Woodsy and pleasant. Smells like ginger, but can vary from supplier to supplier. If you find one with a scent you like, you're going to be hard-pressed to find the same scent anywhere else.

Blending

Blends well with:

- Cedarwood.
- Citrus oils.
- Eucalyptus.
- Floral oils.
- Frankincense.
- Patchouli.
- Sandalwood.
- Spice oils.
- Vetiver.

Therapeutic Properties

Ginger oil is said to have the following therapeutic properties:

- Antispasmodic.
- Aphrodisiac.
- Eases nausea.
- Expectorant.
- Helps ease swelling and pain.
- May improve circulation.
- Stimulates appetite.
- Warming.

Notes

Ginger essential oil can be used for most aromatherapy applications. It's a powerful oil, so be sure to consult a professional prior to adding it to your bag of tricks. Be aware that ginger essential oil contains a high level of hydrocarbons that may damage the lungs.

Ginger Grass Oil

Price

$5 to $15 an ounce.

Derived From

Ginger grass.

Color

Yellow.

Aroma

Green, woody and peppery.

Blending

Blends well with:

- Geranium.
- Hardwood oils.

Therapeutic Properties

Ginger grass oil is said to have the following therapeutic properties:

- Aphrodisiac.
- Improves circulation.
- Opens up respiratory system.
- Reduces stress.
- Uplifting.

Notes

Not to be confused with ginger oil, ginger grass essential oil comes from a flowering grass. It's closer to lemongrass than it is to ginger. It can be used for most aromatherapy purposes, but can irritate the skin, so test it before applying it topically.

Goldenrod Oil

Price

$150 to $200 an ounce.

Derived From

Goldenrod flowers.

Color

Light yellow.

Aroma

Fresh and green. Distinctively strong.

Blending

Blends well with:

- Floral oils.

Therapeutic Properties

Goldenrod oil is said to have the following therapeutic properties:

- Antiallergenic.
- Anti-inflammatory.
- Calming.
- Eases respiratory conditions.
- May help with impotence.
- Reduces stress.
- Relaxing.
- Supports circulatory system.

Notes

Yes, this is the same goldenrod that drives you crazy come allergy season. The oil is generally considered safe for use and nontoxic, but always test in a small area first before application. There are only a select few suppliers that carry this oil and it commands a premium.

Grapefruit Oil

Price

$20 to $100 an ounce.

Derived From

Grapefruit peels.

Color

Yellow.

Aroma

Smells like grapefruit.

Blending

Blends well with:

- Citrus oils.
- Cypress.
- Evergreen oils.
- Frankincense.
- Lavender.

Therapeutic Properties

Grapefruit oil is said to have the following therapeutic properties:

- Antidepressant.
- Antiseptic.
- Astringent.
- Cleanses the body.
- Detoxifying.
- Disinfectant.

- Energizing.

Notes

Grapefruit essential oil can be made from either pink or white grapefruit and can vary widely in price and quality. I prefer pink because it has less of an edge than the white grapefruit oil does. Good grapefruit essential oil works well when diffused and can be added to oil blends for topical application. Grapefruit oil is phototoxic, so avoid exposure to the sun for 24 hours after application.

Helichrysum Oil

Price

$150 to $300 an ounce.

Derived From

Helichrysum flowers.

Color

Light to dark yellow.

Aroma

Sweet and fresh.

Blending

Blends well with:

- Black Pepper.
- Chamomile.
- Citrus oils.
- Clary sage.
- Cypress.
- Floral oils.
- Lavender.
- Rose hip.
- Vetiver.

Therapeutic Properties

Helichrysum oil is said to have the following therapeutic properties:

- Antispasmodic.
- Anticoagulant.

- Antimicrobial.
- Anti-inflammatory.
- Calming.
- Diuretic.
- Eases respiratory problems.
- Emollient.
- May help fade stretch marks.
- Muscle relaxant.
- Relaxing.
- Use to ease the effects of skin problems.
- Thought to ward off cold and flu.

Notes

Helichrysum essential oil works great as a massage oil. This rare and expensive oil can also be used as part of a massage oil blend or it can be added to your natural skin care products.

Hyssop Oil

Price

$70 an ounce.

Derived From

The hyssop plant.

Color

Light yellow to light green.

Aroma

Sweet and earthy.

Blending

Blends well with:

- Cajeput.
- Citrus oils.
- Clary sage.
- Eucalyptus.
- Lavender.
- Myrtle.
- Rosemary.
- Sage.

Therapeutic Properties

Hyssop oil is said to have the following therapeutic properties:

- Alertness.
- Antispasmodic.
- Diuretic.

- Eases respiratory problems.
- Eases stomach problems.
- Fights fatigue.
- PMS relief.
- Relaxing.
- Sedative.
- Sleep disorder relief.

Notes

Hyssop essential oil needs to be used in moderation because it can be neurotoxic in large amounts. Pregnant women and children should avoid exposure to hyssop oil.

Harshingar Oil

Price

$30 an ounce.

Derived From

Night jasmine.

Color

Dark yellow.

Aroma

Exotic.

Blending

Blends well with:

- Floral oils.

Therapeutic Properties

Harshingar oil is said to have the following therapeutic properties:

- Antiviral.
- Antifungal.
- Use to ease vertigo.
- Headache relief.

Notes

Use harshingar essential oil in small amounts. Pregnant women and children should not use harshingar essential oil.

Hiba Oil

Price

$100 an ounce.

Derived From

The Hiba tree, native to Japan.

Color

Yellow.

Aroma

Woody.

Blending

Blends well with:

- Clary sage.
- Evergreen oils.
- Tree oils.
- Ylang ylang.

Therapeutic Properties

Hiba oil is said to have the following therapeutic properties:

- Antibacterial.
- Fight odor.
- Insect repellent.
- Relaxing.
- Used to ease the effects of eczema.

Notes

Hiba oil is especially well-known for its ability to fight bacteria. It's widely considered to be nontoxic and can be used for most aromatherapy purposes.

Inula Oil

Price

$200 to $300 an ounce.

Derived From

The roots of Inula Graveolens plants.

Color

Blue.

Aroma

Floral.

Blending

Inula oil has a unique scent that can be blended with almost anything, but does much better on its own as a standalone scent.

Therapeutic Properties

Inula oil is said to have the following therapeutic properties:

- Antibacterial.
- Calming.
- Decongestant.
- Mucolytic.

Notes

Inula essential oil is great for those with colds and those who are congested. Diffuse the scent and be sure to only add enough of this strong oil to where you can smell it, but it isn't overpowering. Do not apply Inula essential oil topically.

Jasmine Absolute Oil

Price

$100 to $300 an ounce.

Derived From

Jasmine blossoms.

Color

Brown.

Aroma

Floral.

Blending

Blends well with:

- Most other oils.

Therapeutic Properties

Jasmine absolute oil is said to have the following therapeutic properties:

- Antiseptic.
- Antidepressant.
- Antispasmodic.
- Aphrodisiac.
- Expectorant.
- Sedative.
- Uplifting.
- Used to ease the effects of skin problems.
- Used for headaches.

Notes

Jasmine absolute essential oil is strong and must be heavily diluted before use. According to some literature, there may be the risk of an allergic reaction to this oil.

Juniper Berry Oil

Price

$50 an ounce.

Derived From

The berries of juniper trees.

Color

Clear with slight yellow tint.

Aroma

Piney and woody.

Blending

Blends well with:

- Citrus oils.
- Clary sage.
- Lavender.
- Laurel leaf.
- Myrrh.
- Pine.
- Sandalwood.
- Bergamot.

Therapeutic Properties

Juniper berry oil is said to have the following therapeutic properties:

- Anti-inflammatory.
- Antiseptic.
- Calming.

- Clears the mind.
- Diuretic.
- Improves circulation.
- May alleviate acne.
- Moth repellent.
- PMS relief.
- Purifying.
- Relaxing.
- Soothing.

Notes

Juniper berry essential oil lends itself well to most aromatherapy applications. Pregnant women should not use juniper berry oil.

Lavender Oil

Price

$20 to $50 an ounce.

Derived From

Lavender flowers.

Color

Clear.

Aroma

Floral and intricate.

Blending

Blends well with:

- Most other oils. Lavender essential oil is one of the easiest and best oils to use in blends.

Therapeutic Properties

Lavender oil is said to have the following therapeutic properties:

- Anti-inflammatory.
- Balancing.
- Calming.
- Relaxing.
- Thought to help with tissue regeneration.
- Thought to promote wound healing.

Notes

Lavender essential oil is one of the most well-known and versatile essential oils in the world. It's largely nontoxic and it's rare for someone to have an allergic reaction to it. It can be used for all aromatherapy purposes, including direct application of a few drops to the skin. As with all essential oils, test in a small area first, just in case.

Lemon Oil

Price

$10 to $20 an ounce.

Derived From

Lemon peel.

Color

Dark yellow.

Aroma

Smells like lemon.

Blending

Blends well with:

- Other citrus oils.

Therapeutic Properties

Lemon oil is said to have the following therapeutic properties:

- Cleansing.
- Disinfectant.
- Odor control.
- Energizing.
- Uplifting.
- Used to ease the effects of skin problems.

Notes

Lemon essential oil has a scent that almost everyone knows and loves. It smells fresh and clean and is popular in natural household cleaning products. Lemon essential oil can be diffused or diluted and applied topically. It's phototoxic, so avoid sunlight for 24 hours after applying it to the skin. Always test in a small area first to check for an allergic reaction.

Lemongrass Oil

Price

$10 to $15 an ounce.

Derived From

Lemongrass.

Color

Various shades of yellow.

Aroma

Lemony.

Blending

Blends well with:

- Citrus oils.
- Pine.
- Rosemary.

Therapeutic Properties

Lemongrass oil is said to have the following therapeutic properties:

- Antiseptic.
- Antispasmodic.
- Astringent.
- Deodorant.
- Diuretic.
- Headache relief.
- Insect repellent.
- PMS relief.

- Relieves athlete's foot.
- Stimulant.
- Stress relief.

Notes

Lemongrass essential oil is similar to lemon oil and is used for many of the same purposes. It should be avoided by those with glaucoma and those with sensitive skin.

Lime Oil

Price

$10 to $15 an ounce.

Derived From

Lime peels.

Color

Light green.

Aroma

Smells like a lime.

Blending

Blends well with:

- Cedarwood.
- Clary sage.
- Other citrus oils.
- Pine.

Therapeutic Properties

Lime oil is said to have the following therapeutic properties:

- Antibacterial.
- Antiseptic.
- Astringent.
- Cleansing.
- Deodorant.
- Improves circulation.
- Pain relief.

- Pure.
- Renewing.
- Thought to ward off illnesses like the flu and common cold.

Notes

Lime essential oil can be used for most aromatherapy applications. It is known to be phototoxic, so avoid sunlight on the area it was applied to for 24 hours.

Mandarin Oil

Price

$10 to $20 an ounce

Derived From

Mandarin orange peels.

Color

Green.

Aroma

Sweet orange.

Blending

Blends well with:

- Citrus oils.
- Lavender.
- Spicy oils.

Therapeutic Properties

Mandarin oil is said to have the following therapeutic properties:

- Calming.
- Heals skin.
- Relaxing.
- Relieves stomach issues.
- Soothing.
- Used for those with insomnia.

Notes

Mandarin essential oil is one of the milder essential oils and is considered safe for most aromatherapy applications. It's one of the few essential oils deemed safe for use with children, but always consult with a medical professional before use.

Manuka Oil

Price

$40 to $50 an ounce.

Derived From

The Manuka tree.

Color

Clear.

Aroma

Woody.

Blending

Blends well with:

- Chamomile.
- Floral oils.
- Spice oils.

Therapeutic Properties

Manuka oil is said to have the following therapeutic properties:

- Anti-inflammatory.
- Heals skin.
- Relieves cold and flu symptoms.

Notes

Manuka essential oil can be used for most aromatherapy purposes. Manuka essential oil is relatively unknown and there hasn't been a lot of research done into whether or not it's completely safe. Be aware that manuka essential oil contains a high level of hydrocarbons that may damage the lungs.

Marjoram Oil

Price

$10 to $20 an ounce.

Derived From

Marjoram herb.

Color

Slight yellow tint.

Aroma

Herbaceous and campherous.

Blending

Blends well with:

- Eucalyptus.
- Hardwood oils.
- Lavender.

Therapeutic Properties

Marjoram oil is said to have the following therapeutic properties:

- Antibacterial.
- Antifungal.
- Anti-inflammatory.
- Eases the effects of respiratory problems.
- Relieves muscle pains and cramping.
- Sedative.
- Wards off infection.

Notes

Marjoram essential oil is a diverse oil that can be diffused or used in various oil blends and applied topically.

May Chang (Litsea) Oil

Price

$6 to $10 an ounce.

Derived From

May Chang trees.

Color

Dark yellow.

Aroma

Fresh and lemony.

Blending

Blends well with:

- Chamomile.
- Grapeseed.
- Hazelnut.

Therapeutic Properties

May Chang oil is said to have the following therapeutic properties:

- Aids digestion.
- Antidepressant.
- Antimicrobial.
- Antiseptic.
- Cooling.
- Good for skin.
- May help with excessive perspiration.
- Soothing.

Notes

May Chang essential oil can be used for most aromatherapy purposes, but should be avoided by those with glaucoma and those with sensitive skin.

Melissa (Lemon Balm) Oil

Price

$100 to $300 an ounce.

Derived From

Melissa plant.

Color

Light yellow.

Aroma

Sweet citrus.

Blending

Blends well with:

- Basil.
- Chamomile.
- Citrus oils.
- Lavender.
- Rose.

Therapeutic Properties

Melissa oil is said to have the following therapeutic properties:

- Antidepressant.
- Antifungal.
- Calming.
- Eases tension.
- May help lower blood pressure.
- May help with migraines.

- Sedative.

Notes

Melissa essential oil is also known as lemon balm oil. It works great in diffusers and oil blends, but can be a little tough on the skin when applied topically. Always dilute heavily and test on a small area before use.

Mountain Savory Oil

Price

$50 to $100 an ounce.

Derived From

Mountain savory plant.

Color

Dark yellow.

Aroma

Fresh.

Blending

Blends well with:

- Spice oils.

Therapeutic Properties

Mountain savory oil is said to have the following therapeutic properties:

- Antibacterial.
- Antifungal.
- Anti-parasitic.
- Antiseptic.
- Boosts the immune system.
- General tonic.
- May stimulate the adrenal gland.

Notes

Mountain savory is relatively hard to find and is only available through a handful of suppliers. It has powerful antiseptic qualities and is a good choice for diluting and applying topically or it can be diffused. Women who are pregnant should avoid this oil.

Myrhh Oil

Price

$75 to $100 an ounce.

Derived From

The resin of the myrrh tree.

Color

Golden yellow.

Aroma

Warm and floral.

Blending

Blends well with:

- Floral oils.
- Frankincense.
- Hardwood oils.
- Patchouli.
- Spice oils.

Therapeutic Properties

Myrrh oil is said to have the following therapeutic properties:

- Anti-inflammatory.
- Antiseptic.
- Assists with kidney function.
- Improves circulation.
- May reduce wrinkles.
- Meditative.

- Mellowing.
- Oral health.
- Spiritual.
- Used to treat skin conditions.
- Uterine stimulant.

Notes

Myrrh essential oil can be toxic when ingested or used in large amounts. Use it sparingly with your products and massage oil blends for best results. Pregnant women should avoid myrrh.

Myrtle Oil

Price

$20 to $40 an ounce.

Derived From

Leaves and twigs of the myrtle tree.

Color

Brown.

Aroma

Campherous. Reminiscent of eucalyptus.

Blending

Blends well with:

- Clary sage.
- Clove.
- Eucalyptus.
- Mint oils.
- Spicy oils.

Therapeutic Properties

Myrtle oil is said to have the following therapeutic properties:

- Antiseptic.
- Astringent.
- Expectorant.
- Respiratory health.
- Said by some to help ease the transition away from addictions.

- Skin care.
- Used for acne.
- Used for respiratory problems.
- Used for sore throats.

Notes

There are two basic varieties of myrtle essential oil, green and red. The green oil is made from the leaves and twigs of the myrtle tree and is the oil you want to use for aromatherapy purposes. It can be diluted and applied topically or it can be diffused. Always test on a small area of skin first.

P a g e | **241**

Neroli (Orange Flower) Oil

Price

$400 an ounce.

Derived From

Orange blossoms.

Color

Brown.

Aroma

Floral, with a hint of citrus.

Blending

Blends well with:

- Citrus oils.
- Floral oils.
- Sandalwood.

Therapeutic Properties

Neroli oil is said to have the following therapeutic properties:

- Antibacterial.
- Antidepressant.
- Antiseptic.
- Antispasmodic.
- Aphrodisiac.
- Deodorant.
- Disinfectant.
- Emollient.

- Relaxing.
- Sedative.

Notes

This is an expensive oil because the blossoms are difficult to harvest and distill. Neroli essential oil is primarily used in high-end perfumes, but it can be used for aromatherapy purposes as well. This oil is generally considered to be safe, but it is phototoxic, so avoid exposure to the sun for 24 hours after applying it topically. As with all essential oils, always test it on a small area first.

Niaouli Oil

Price

$5 to $10 an ounce.

Derived From

Niaouli trees.

Color

Clear yellow.

Aroma

Deeply earthy.

Blending

Blends well with:

- Coriander.
- Eucalyptus.
- Evergreen oils.
- Lavender.
- Lemon.
- Lime.
- Tea tree.

Therapeutic Properties

Niaouli oil is said to have the following therapeutic properties:

- Analgesic.
- Antibacterial.
- Antiseptic.
- Benefits immune system.

- Decongestant.
- Energizing.
- Expectorant.
- Insect repellent.
- Thought to remove blemishes.

Notes

Niaouli essential oil is primarily used for its antiseptic qualities and can be used for most aromatherapy applications.

Nutmeg Oil

Price

$10 to $20 an ounce.

Derived From

Nutmeg seeds.

Color

Clear.

Aroma

Spicy. Smell like nutmeg, only stronger.

Blending

Blends well with:

- Lime.
- Spice oils.
- Sweet orange.

Therapeutic Properties

Nutmeg oil is said to have the following therapeutic properties:

- Antioxidant.
- Antiseptic.
- Aphrodisiac.
- Improves circulation.
- Stimulant.
- Used for stomach problems.

Notes

Nutmeg essential oil can be toxic in larger amounts. Use under the supervision of an aromatherapy specialist and be sure to consult with your physician before use.

Oak Moss Oil

Price

$75 to $100 an ounce.

Derived From

Oak moss.

Color

Brown.

Aroma

Mossy lavender.

Blending

Blends well with:

- Citrus oils.
- Lavender.

Therapeutic Properties

Oak moss oil is said to have the following therapeutic properties:

- Aids with respiratory problems.
- Expectorant.

Notes

Oak moss oil should be heavily diluted before use. The heavy, mossy scent will overpower other scents if you use more than a drop or two.

Orange Oil (Sweet)

Price

$8 to $15 an ounce.

Derived From

Orange peels.

Color

Orange.

Aroma

Smells like oranges.

Blending

Blends well with:

- Most essential oils.

Therapeutic Properties

Orange oil is said to have the following therapeutic properties:

- Antidepressant.
- Anti-inflammatory.
- Antiseptic.
- Antispasmodic.
- Aphrodisiac.
- Calming.
- Diuretic.
- Good for skin.
- May combat wrinkles.

Notes

Orange essential oil is generally considered safe for aromatherapy use, but may be phototoxic. Just to be safe, I'd avoid exposing the area where it's applied to the sun for at least 24 hours.

Oregano Oil

Price

$15 to $20 an ounce.

Derived From

Oregano.

Color

Light yellow.

Aroma

Smells like oregano, only stronger.

Blending

Blends well with:

- Chamomile.
- Lavender.
- Wood oils.

Therapeutic Properties

Oregano oil is said to have the following therapeutic properties:

- Antiviral.
- Antifungal.
- Antibacterial.
- Anti-parasitic.
- May ease PMS symptoms.
- Relaxing.
- Sedative.
- Stress relief.

- Used to relieve digestive problems.
- Used to relieve respiratory problems.
- Used to relieve swelling.

Notes

Oregano essential oil is generally helpful in small amounts, but can be an irritant when larger amounts are used. Always dilute heavily and test in a small area before applying topically.

Palmarosa Oil

Price

$15 an ounce.

Derived From

Palmarosa plant.

Color

Clear, with a slight yellow tint.

Aroma

Floral and clean.

Blending

Blends well with:

- Citrus oils.
- Spice oils.

Therapeutic Properties

Palmarosa oil is said to have the following therapeutic properties:

- Antibacterial.
- Antifungal.
- Antiseptic.
- Antiviral.
- Helps the user focus.
- May fade wrinkles.
- Stimulant.
- Used to ease the effects of skin conditions.
- Used to help stomach problems.

Notes

Palmarosa oil is so much like Rose Geranium oil that some sources claim it's the same thing. It isn't, but it's close enough that the confusion really doesn't matter. Palmarosa oil can be used for most aromatherapy purposes, but lends itself particularly well to diffusion because of its pleasant scent.

Palo Santo Oil

Price

$40 to $50 an ounce.

Derived From

The wood of the Palo Santo tree.

Color

Clear to yellow.

Aroma

Woody, with a hint of citrus.

Blending

Blends well with:

- Frankincense.
- Geranium.
- Lemon.
- Wood oils.

Therapeutic Properties

Palo Santo oil is said to have the following therapeutic properties:

- Calming.
- Focus.
- Insect repellent.
- Relaxing.
- Relieves muscle tension and pain.
- Thought to fight cancer.
- Used to ease the effects of respiratory problems.

Notes

Palo Santo oil works well when diffused. Palo Santo oils is a known dermal irritant, so avoid applying it topically. If you do decide to try it, dilute it heavily and test on a small area first.

Parsley Seed Oil

Price

$30 to $40 an ounce.

Derived From

Parsley seeds.

Color

Clear yellow.

Aroma

Herbaceous. Smells similar to parsley, but stronger.

Blending

Blends well with:

- Herb oils.
- Rose.
- Spice oils.

Therapeutic Properties

Parsley seed oil is said to have the following therapeutic properties:

- Detoxifies the body.
- Encourages menstruation.
- May lower blood pressure.
- Used to aid menstrual cramping.

Notes

Parsley seed oils contains chemical compounds that are toxic to the organs of the human body and is capable of causing pregnant women to abort. You should only use this oil with the approval of your doctor and it should be done under the care of an aromatherapy specialist.

Patchouli Oil

Price

$20 an ounce.

Derived From

Patchouli leaves.

Color

Amber.

Aroma

Unique. Deep and woody.

Blending

Blends well with:

- Most other oils.

Therapeutic Properties

Patchouli oil is said to have the following therapeutic properties:

- Antidepressant.
- Anti-inflammatory.
- Aphrodisiac.
- Astringent.
- Calming.
- Decongestant.
- Deodorant.
- Grounding.
- Insect repellent.
- Promotes regrowth of skin cells.

- Soothes skin.
- Stimulant.

Notes

Patchouli essential oil is one of the more diverse oils and can be used for most aromatherapy applications. It takes a while to get used to the smell, but it grows on you and soon you won't be able to do without your patchouli oil. Patchouli oil is one of a few oils that smell better as they age.

Peppermint Oil

Price

$5 to $15 an ounce.

Derived From

Peppermint.

Color

Clear yellow.

Aroma

Strong mint aroma.

Blending

Blends well with:

- Citrus oils.
- Wood oils.

Therapeutic Properties

Peppermint oil is said to have the following therapeutic properties:

- Aphrodisiac.
- Cooling.
- Eases aches and pains.

Notes

Peppermint essential oil is strong and can cause a number of issues if not administered properly. Consult with a professional before beginning use of peppermint oil.

Petitgrain Oil

Price

$15 an ounce.

Derived From

Bitter orange tree leaves.

Color

Clear yellow.

Aroma

Citrus, woody and clean.

Blending

Blends well with:

- Citrus oils.
- Floral oils.
- Wood oils.

Therapeutic Properties

Petitgrain oil is said to have the following therapeutic properties:

- Antidepressant.
- Antiseptic.
- Calming.
- Concentration.
- Deodorant.
- Relaxing.
- Skin care.
- Stimulant.

- Stress relief.

Notes

Petitgrain is generally considered safe for most aromatherapy applications. If you plant on applying it topically, always dilute and test in a small area first.

Pine Oil

Price

$5 to $10 an ounce.

Derived From

Pine needles.

Color

Clear yellow.

Aroma

Piney and woody.

Blending

Blends well with:

- Camphoric oils.
- Wood oils.

Therapeutic Properties

Pine oil is said to have the following therapeutic properties:

- Analgesic.
- Anti-inflammatory.
- Calming.
- Decongestant.
- Eases the effects of respiratory conditions.
- Improves circulation.
- May help with arthritis and rheumatism.
- Stress relief.

Notes

Pine oil can be used for some aromatherapy applications, but there is a chance it may react with your skin. Always dilute and test in a small area first. Consult with an aromatherapy specialist prior to beginning use of pine oil as it can be a mucous membrane irritant and can be somewhat toxic if ingested.

Ravensara Oil

Price

$10 an ounce.

Derived From

Ravensara leaves.

Color

Light yellow.

Aroma

Medicinal and slightly campherous.

Blending

Blends well with:

- Eucalyptus.
- Wood oils.

Therapeutic Properties

Ravensara oil is said to have the following therapeutic properties:

- Antibacterial.
- Antifungal.
- Antiseptic.
- Is used to ease athlete's foot.
- May ease respiratory problems.

Notes

Ravensara essential oil is believed to be safe for most people to use, but there is relatively little documentation available on this oil. Avoid it when pregnant and test your tolerance by using small amounts at first.

Rose Oil

Price

$300 to $500 an ounce.

Derived From

Rose petals.

Color

Red or yellow.

Aroma

Floral.

Blending

Blends well with:

- Floral oils.
- Frankincense.

Therapeutic Properties

Rose oil is said to have the following therapeutic properties:

- Anti-inflammatory.
- Aphrodisiac.
- Astringent.
- Calming.
- Comforting.
- Moisturizes skin.
- Relaxing.
- Sensual.
- Stress relief.

Notes

Rose oil comes in two forms: absolute or otto. The otto is the better of the two, but it comes at a premium. Absolute can be used for most aromatherapy purposes. Go with the otto if you're using your rose oil to help ease the effects of skin conditions.

Rose oil is expensive, but a little oil goes a long way. It can be diffused, but you're better off saving it for sensual massage oil blends. Always dilute and test in a small area first, but rose oil is generally considered one of the safer oils to apply topically in an oil blend.

Rosemary Oil

Price

$5 to $10 an ounce.

Derived From

Rosemary herb.

Color

Clear to yellow.

Aroma

Strong and herbal.

Blending

Blends well with:

- Citrus oils.
- Frankincense.
- Peppermint.
- Spice oils.

Therapeutic Properties

Rosemary oil is said to have the following therapeutic properties:

- Antidepressant.
- Antimicrobial.
- Antiseptic.
- Balancing.
- Calming.
- Nourishes skin.
- Stimulant.

- Uplifting.
- Used to ease respiratory issues.
- Used to ease skin conditions.

Notes

Avoid rosemary essential oil if you have high blood pressure. It should also be avoided by pregnant women and those with epilepsy.

Rosewood Oil

Price

$50 an ounce.

Derived From

Rosewood trees, which are endangered. Only buy this oil from suppliers who use sustainable sources.

Color

Light yellow.

Aroma

Earthy and floral.

Blending

Blends well with:

- Most other oils.

Therapeutic Properties

Rosewood oil is said to have the following therapeutic properties:

- Antidepressant.
- Aphrodisiac.
- Stress relief.
- Used for impotence.
- Used to help ease respiratory conditions.
- Used to help with common cold and flu.
- Used to promote skin health.

Notes

Rosewood essential oil is generally considered safe for most aromatherapy purposes. As with all essential oils, dilute it and test it in a small area prior to application.

Sage Oil

Price

$15 to $20 an ounce.

Derived From

Any of a number of different varieties of sage plants.

Color

Light yellow.

Aroma

Herbaceous and campherous.

Blending

Blends well with:

- Floral oils.
- Spice oils.

Therapeutic Properties

Sage oil is said to have the following therapeutic properties:

- Antimicrobial.
- Antiviral.
- Expectorant.
- Improves circulation.
- May fade scars.
- May promote healing of wounds.
- Stimulating.

Notes

Sage essential oil is powerful stuff. So powerful that some experts recommend avoiding it entirely because of its high thujone content. If you decide to use this oil, do so under the supervision of an aromatherapy professional and be sure to dilute it to less than 1%. Do not take this oil internally.

Sandalwood Oil

Price

$75 to $300 an ounce.

Derived From

Sandalwood heartwood and roots. There are a number of types of sandalwood that this oil is made from.

Color

Clear, with a slight yellow tint.

Aroma

Woody, with a hint of floral.

Blending

Blends well with:

- Citrus oils.
- Frankincense.
- Spice oils.
- Wood oils.

Therapeutic Properties

Sandalwood oil is said to have the following therapeutic properties:

- Aids with circulation.
- Antifungal.
- Antiseptic.
- Astringent.
- Emollient.
- Expectorant.

- May be an aphrodisiac.
- Stimulant.
- Used for insomnia.
- Used to ease skin conditions.

Notes

Sandalwood trees are rare and have been severely depleted, which is why the cost of this oil is on the rise. It's a popular oil and can be used for most aromatherapy applications.

Spearmint Oil

Price

$10 an ounce.

Derived From

Spearmint plant.

Color

Clear yellow.

Aroma

Minty. More refined than peppermint.

Blending

Blends well with:

- Most other oils.

Therapeutic Properties

Spearmint oil is said to have the following therapeutic properties:

- Antibacterial.
- Antiseptic.
- Diuretic.
- Expectorant.
- Headache relief.
- Skin care.
- Stimulant.
- Stress relief.

Notes

Spearmint essential oil is one of the milder mint oils and can be used when you want to add a hint of mint to your oil blends or products. It's still a mucous membrane irritant in large amounts, but not as much so as peppermint or the stronger oils. Always dilute and test in a small area before applying topically.

Spikenard Oil

Price

$30 to $70 an ounce.

Derived From

Roots of the spikenard plant.

Color

Deep yellow.

Aroma

Oriental. Spicy.

Blending

Blends well with:

- Evergreen oils.
- Floral oils.
- Spice oils.

Therapeutic Properties

Spikenard oil is said to have the following therapeutic properties:

- Antibacterial.
- Antifungal.
- Anti-inflammatory.
- Deodorant.
- Laxative.
- Sedative.
- Skin care.

Notes

Spikenard essential oil is generally considered safe for most aromatherapy applications. Always dilute and test in a small area before applying it topically.

Spruce Oil

Price

$15 to $20 an ounce.

Derived From

Spruce needles and twigs.

Color

Clear.

Aroma

Piney and earthy.

Blending

Blends well with:

- Cedarwood.
- Lavender.
- Pine.
- Rosemary .

Therapeutic Properties

Spruce oil is said to have the following therapeutic properties:

- Antiseptic.
- Calming.
- Expectorant.
- Relief of aches and pains.
- Respiratory health.
- Uplifting.

Notes

Spruce essential oil is one of the lighter evergreen oils. It can be used for most aromatherapy applications. Always dilute heavily and test a small area before application.

Tangerine Oil

Price

$10 to $20 an ounce.

Derived From

Tangerine peels.

Color

Green.

Aroma

Citrus. Lighter than orange oil.

Blending

Blends well with:

- Black pepper.
- Cinnamon.
- Frankincense.
- Juniper.
- Myrrh.
- Patchouli.
- Rose.

Therapeutic Properties

Tangerine oil is said to have the following therapeutic properties:

- Calming.
- Relieves tension.
- Sedative.
- Skin care.

- Used for insomnia.

Notes

Tangerine essential oil may be phototoxic. Stay out of the sun for at least 24 hours after you apply the oil. Tangerine oil can be used for most aromatherapy applications.

Tea Tree Oil

Price

$10 to $150 an ounce.

Derived From

Tea tree leaves and twigs.

Color

Clear with a yellow tint.

Aroma

Warm and spicy.

Blending

Blends well with:

- Campherous oils.
- Citrus oils.
- Lavender.

Therapeutic Properties

Tea tree oil is said to have the following therapeutic properties:

- Antibacterial.
- Antibiotic.
- Antifungal.
- Anti-inflammatory.
- Antiseptic.
- Antiviral.
- Expectorant.
- Insect repellent.

- Skin care.
- Stimulant.

Notes

The price of tea tree essential oil varies greatly, depending on the quality and rarity of the type of tea tree it's harvested from. The quality also varies greatly. Check with the supplier to see what the type of tea tree essential oil you're thinking about buying can be used for.

Thyme Oil

Price

$20 to $30 an ounce.

Derived From

Thyme.

Color

Brown.

Aroma

Herbaceous and spicy.

Blending

Blends well with:

- Campherous oils.
- Citrus oils.

Therapeutic Properties

Thyme oil is said to have the following therapeutic properties:

- Germicidal.
- Improves circulation.
- Relaxing.
- Skin care.
- Used for cold relief.
- Warming.

Notes

Thyme essential oil is only to be used in small amounts and must be heavily diluted before use. Always consult with a healthcare and an aromatherapy professional before use.

Turmeric Oil

Price

$5 to $10 an ounce.

Derived From

Turmeric plant.

Color

Yellow to orange.

Aroma

Spicy and woody.

Blending

Blends well with:

- Spice oils.

Therapeutic Properties

Turmeric essential oil is said to have the following therapeutic properties:

- Antiseptic.
- Balancing.
- Relaxing.
- Skin care.

Notes

Turmeric essential oil can be a dermal and mucous membrane irritant when used in large amounts. Consult with a medical and an aromatherapy professional before use.

Vanilla Oil

Price

$15 to $150 an ounce.

Derived From

Vanilla beans.

Color

Brown.

Aroma

Vanilla.

Blending

Blends well with:

- Most essential oils.

Therapeutic Properties

Vanilla oil is said to have the following therapeutic properties:

- Aphrodisiac.
- Calming.
- Relaxing.
- Skin care.
- Stimulating.

Notes

Vanilla essential oil has a pleasant scent that's familiar to almost everyone. It varies widely in price. You're better off going with one of the more expensive oils that's been CO_2-

distilled, as opposed to one of the cheaper solvent-extracted oils.

Vetiver Oil

Price

$25 to $50 an ounce.

Derived From

Vetiver grass.

Color

Brown.

Aroma

Herbaceous and smoky.

Blending

Blends well with:

- Lavender.
- Patchouli.
- Ylang ylang.

Therapeutic Properties

Vetiver oil is said to have the following therapeutic properties:

- Calming.
- Relaxing.
- Skin care.
- Slows heart rate.
- Soothes muscle aches and pains.
- Uplifting.

Notes

Vetiver essential oil is like a fine wine, in that it gets better with age. It can be used for most aromatherapy applications. As with all oils, dilute and test on a small patch of skin before applying topically.

Wintergreen Oil

Price

$10 to $20 an ounce.

Derived From

Wintergreen shrubs.

Color

Light yellow.

Aroma

Strong mint.

Blending

Blends well with:

- Lavender.
- Mint oils.
- Oregano.
- Thyme.
- Vanilla.
- Ylang ylang.

Therapeutic Properties

Wintergreen oil is said to have the following therapeutic properties:

- Anti-inflammatory.
- Antiseptic.
- Calming.
- Deodorant.
- Pain relief.

- Stimulant.

Notes

Wintergreen essential oil contains methyl salicylate, which is similar to aspirin in make-up. This oil should only be used under the supervision of a medical professional.

Yarrow Oil

Price

$30 to $50 an ounce

Derived From

Yarrow herb.

Color

Blue.

Aroma

Herbaceous and spicy.

Blending

Blends well with:

- Frankincense.
- Myrrh.

Therapeutic Properties

Yarrow oil is said to have the following therapeutic properties:

- Balancing.
- Skin care.
- Used to promote healing of minor wounds.

Notes

Yarrow essential oil is thought to be non-toxic in small amounts, but can be toxic when larger dosages are used. Always dilute heavily before use and test in a small area before applying topically.

Ylang Ylang Oil

Price

$25 to $150 an ounce.

Derived From

Ylang ylang flowers.

Color

Clear yellow.

Aroma

Exotic and sweet.

Blending

Blends well with:

- Most other oils.

Therapeutic Properties

Ylang ylang oil is said to have the following therapeutic properties:

- Antidepressant.
- Anti-infectious.
- Antiseptic.
- Aphrodisiac.
- Euphoric.
- Sedative.

Notes

Ylang ylang oil varies greatly in price based on how many times the oil has been distilled. The more times it's put through the process, the more beneficial ingredients it will have.

Potentially Dangerous Essential Oils

Let me begin this chapter by stating that all essential oils are powerful enough to do harm if used in the wrong manner. It's recommend that you begin your journey under the watchful eye of both your physician and an aromatherapy professional in order to make sure you make smart choices.

The essential oils listed in this chapter are known to be especially hazardous when used in the wrong way. I want to make it clear that this list is not a complete list of all the oils and all the associated potential complications, and just because an oil or a complication didn't make the list, that doesn't automatically mean it's safe to use freely and without concern.

There may be complications that I missed during my research for this book and there may be complications that haven't yet been associated with a particular oil. Take the information for what it's worth. It's a good start into understanding which oils are dangerous, but it isn't a complete encyclopedia. To my knowledge, a complete database of the potential hazards doesn't exist.

It's also important to realize that an essential oil that's generally considered safe to use can be made unsafe during the distillation process. This is especially true when solvents and chemicals are used because those solvents and chemicals can and often do find their way into essential oils.

There's also the possibility of an allergic reaction. Make sure you always test your essential oils by diluting them heavily the first time you use them. It's preferable to have an allergic reaction in a small area that's inconspicuous than it is to have a reaction spread over a rather large visible area. Trust me on that one. Learn from my mistakes.

Most oils need to be diluted before they're applied topically. Applying oil at full strength is a good way to "burn" your skin, similar to the type of burn you'd get if exposed to a caustic chemical. There are a select few oils that can be applied neat, but you need to know what you're doing before attempting to apply them in this manner and should proceed with extreme caution. Be aware that not everyone has the same level of tolerance for an oil. What works for you or a neighbor may result in an adverse reaction for the next guy.

The same thing goes for diffusion of essential oil. Keep the amount of oil you're using for dispersion to a minimum until you see how your body tolerates it. You don't have to come in direct contact with an oil for it to irritate your lungs, nose and eyes.

The following essential oils are known to be hazardous in one form or another. You may notice some of these oils aren't in the previous chapter. That's because the dangers of using the excluded oils far outweigh the benefits and you should avoid them unless you're using them under the careful guidance of a professional. Even then, I'd be leery of using some of these oils. There are probably far safer alternatives that don't pose the same risks.

Anise Oil

Anise oil contains *anethol* and trace amounts of *methyl chavicol*, which can destroy the nervous system and lead to paralysis. Anise oil is toxic enough that it should be avoided for aromatherapy purposes unless used for a specific reason under the strict supervision of a medical professional.

Armoise Oil

Armoise oil contains high levels of thujones, which are toxic to the body if ingested. Only use this oil under the supervision of an aromatherapy professional and with the approval of your doctor.

Benzoin Oil

Contains allergens that are known to cause sensitization. Benzoin oil is removed from resin using a solvent, which can leave trace amounts of harmful chemicals behind in the oil. It's best to avoid benzoin essential oil altogether.

Bitter Almond Oil

Bitter almond oil contains both *cyanide* and *benzaldehyde*. Both are known toxic substances that are extremely toxic if ingested in anything but the smallest of amounts. A capful of oil could be deadly. Bitter almond oil should only be used under the strict supervision of a professional.

Birch Tar Oil

This oil contains polynuclear hydrocarbons that are carcinogenic. Don't use birch tar oil for aromatherapy purposes.

Birch Oil

Sweet birch oil contains methyl salicylate, which is converted to salicylic acid once it enters the body. Extended use can cause permanent liver damage. Be aware that methyl salicylate is readily absorbed through the skin, so topical application can result in elevated levels of salicylic acid in the body.

Boldo Leaf Oil

Boldo leaf oil contains *ascaridole*, a substance that's toxic and can induce convulsions when small amounts are taken orally. This oil should be avoided at all costs.

Brown or Yellow Camphor Oil

These oils have been banned in some countries because they contain *safrole*, which is a known carcinogen. White camphor is a moderately safer alternative.

Cade Oil

While cade oil is still in use by some aromatherapy practitioners, it contains compounds that are suspected carcinogens. It's best to avoid using cade oil for aromatherapy purposes.

Calamus Oil

This oil contains *asarone* and is potentially carcinogenic and toxic when ingested. Use only under the strict supervision of a professional and with the approval of your doctor.

Camphor Oil

Camphor oil can be fatal if even a small amount is ingested. It's also believed to cause lung problems when inhaled in large amounts. To top things off, it's a dermal irritant. Do not use camphor oil for aromatherapy purposes.

White camphor oil is marginally safer and can be effective in certain applications, but should only be used under the watchful eye of an aromatherapy professional.

Cinnamon Bark Oil

Cinnamon bark oil can elicit a strong dermal reaction and can cause sensitization issues. It's still in use in aromatherapy, but should only be used under the supervision of a professional and with the approval of your doctor.

Costus Oil

Costus oil is a strong dermal irritant. It's used to scent some perfumes, but should be avoided for aromatherapy purposes.

Croton Oil

Croton oil contains the compound *phorbol*, which is a blistering agent that causes the skin to blister and peel. Do not use croton oil for aromatherapy purposes.

Elecampene Oil

Elecampene oil is a potential dermal irritant that can cause sensitization of the skin. This oil is generally avoided when it comes to aromatherapy.

Fig Leaf Absolute

It's recommended by the International Fragrance Association that fig leaf absolute is avoided because of its phototoxicity and the potential for dermal irritation.

Horseradish Oil

If you've ever eaten horseradish, you've tasted allyl isothiocyanate. It's what gives horseradish its distinctive bitter taste. It's a dermal irritant capable of inducing severe reactions. In fact, it's one of the compounds used to make gases used in war. Steer clear of horseradish oil.

Massoia Bark Oil

Massoia bark oil is a dermal irritant that can cause flushing and skin sensitization. Avoid this oil for aromatherapy purposes.

Melilotus Oil

Melilotus oil contains high levels of coumarin, which can be toxic to the internal organs when taken orally. The coumarin in this oil may be absorbed into the bloodstream when applied topically, so it's best to avoid melilotus oil completely.

Mustard Oil

Allyl isothiocyanate is present in mustard oil in high enough levels to make it a strong dermal irritant. Avoid this oil for aromatherapy purposes.

Ocotea Oil

This oil is high in *safrole*, which is one of the key ingredients used to create the recreational drug ecstasy. Safrole is a known carcinogen, so steer clear of this oil.

Oils Containing High Levels of Hydrocarbons

The following oils contain high levels of hydrocarbons and are thought to damage the lungs upon being taken in:

- Cedarwood.
- Ginger.
- Manuka.

Oils Containing Methyleugenol

Methyleugenol has been shown in a lab setting to be a carcinogenic compound when used in large amounts. It may be safe to use oils containing this compound in tiny amounts, but they need to be diluted to less than one tenth of one percent for topical application and less than 2% for diffusion.

The following oils are known to contain methyleugenol:

- Allspice (large amounts).
- Armoise (small amounts).
- Basil (amount varies depending on type of basil used).
- Bay laurel (large amounts).
- Bay (large amounts).
- Carrot (none at all to small amounts).
- Citronella (none at all to small amounts).
- Melaleuca (large amounts).
- Myrtle (can have large amounts).
- Oregano (large amounts).
- Ravensara (large amounts).
- Rose (varies).
- Tarragon (large amounts).
- Tea tree (large amounts).
- Ylang ylang (varies, but usually isn't present).

Oils Containing Thymol

Thymol is believed to be helpful in small dosages, but can be harmful in larger amounts. Dilute oils containing thymol heavily. Keep oils that contain thymol away from children and pregnant women.

The following essential oils contain thymol:

- Ajowan.
- Aljwain.
- Bergamot.

- Oregano.
- Thyme.

Parsley Seed Oil

Aromatherapy professionals do occasionally use this oil because of its detoxification abilities. If it's used incorrectly, it can be toxic and should be avoided unless it's being used under the close scrutiny of a professional and with the approval of your doctor.

Phototoxic Oils

While we touched upon a number of oils that are thought to be phototoxic in the previous chapter, it doesn't hurt to list them in one place. *Phototoxic oils* cause the skin to become unnaturally sensitive to sunlight. Extreme phototoxic reactions can lead to burns similar to those you'd get from a bad sunburn.

The following oils are thought to be phototoxic:

- Angelica root oil.
- Bergamot oil.
- Cumin oil.
- Fig leaf oil.
- Most citrus oils.
- Parsley leaf oil.
- Rue oil.
- Tagetes oil.
- Tansy oil.
- Verbena oil.

Pine Oil

Pine oil is a strong oil that can irritate the skin and mucous membranes. It can cause shortness of breath and breathing problems when used in larger doses. Taking pine oil internally isn't recommended because it can be toxic to the internal organs. Use pine oil with caution and be sure to test it and heavily dilute it.

Rue Oil

This is bad stuff and should never be used for aromatherapy. It's phototoxic, a strong dermal irritant and can sensitize the skin.

Santolina Oil

Santolina essential oil is another oil that's high in safrole and needs to be avoided.

Sassafras Oil

Sassafras oil has been all but banned in the European Union and by the FDA in the United States because of its carcinogenic properties. Do not use it for aromatherapy purposes, as it can be toxic if administered incorrectly.

Southernwood Oil

Southernwood oil contains thujone, which is toxic to the liver. Don't use this oil for aromatherapy purposes.

Tansy Oil

Tansy essential oil contains thujone, which is lethal if even a small amount is ingested. Blue Tansy oil may be safer, but there is contradicting information out there regarding its safety. Most sources say it's non-toxic.

Thuja Oil

Thuja oil also contains elevated levels of thujone and should be avoided for aromatherapy purposes.

Tonka Bean Oil

Contain coumarin, which is toxic when ingested.

Turpentine Oil

Turpentine is used in paint thinners and nail polish removers because of its caustic qualities. Turpentine essential oil is strong stuff that shouldn't be used for aromatherapy because it can burn the skin and is toxic when ingested orally.

Verbena Oil

Pure verbena oil is a powerful dermal irritant. Synthetic oil doesn't cause the same problems, but also doesn't offer much other than the scent.

Wintergreen Oil

Wintergreen oil contains methyl salicylate, which is converted to salicylic acid once it enters the body. Extended use can cause permanent liver damage. Be aware that methyl salicylate is readily absorbed through the skin, so topical application can result in elevated levels of salicylic acid in the body.

Wormseed Oil

This oil is so toxic that it's been banned for sale in the UK. Don't use it for aromatherapy applications.

Fake Essential Oils

There are a number of counterfeit essential oils on the market today. At times, even the people selling them have been duped into believing they're real, when the oil is actually a synthetic blend or has been heavily diluted.

This practice is troubling on multiple levels.

Most people use essential oils because of their therapeutic value. The fake oils have little to no value when it comes to improving one's health and easing the effects of certain medical conditions. Even more troubling is the fact that you never know what's going to be in the fake oil. People who are capable of selling fake oil often have no qualms as to what they put in the oil to make it appear real. You could potentially be putting a harmful chemical cocktail on your skin or into your body that could be doing more harm than good.

The following list identifies essential oils that are commonly faked. If you do find one of these as a real oil, it's going to cost you a pretty penny because of its rarity:

- Agarwood.
- Almond.
- Aloe Vera apple.
- Ambergis.
- Apricot.
- Banana.
- Brown sugar.
- Carnation.
- Cherry and cherry blossom.

- Coconut.
- Fig.
- Hazelnut.
- Honeysuckle.
- Hyacinth.
- Kiwi.
- Lettuce.
- Lily.
- Lotus.
- Mango.
- Melissa.
- Musk.
- Papaya.
- Peach.
- Pear.
- Pineapple.
- Plum.
- Sunflower.
- Tuberose.
- Vanilla.
- Various berry oils (blackberry, blueberry, strawberry, etc.).
- Various melon oils (watermelon, honeydew, etc.).

It isn't uncommon for manufacturers to fake some of the more common oils like frankincense, myrrh and sandalwood as well. Always buy from a reputable supplier and keep an eye out for oils that don't look, smell or feel right.

Are Essential Oils Safe for Pregnant and Nursing Women?

In a word, maybe.

While there are some essential oils like sage oil and savin oil that contain substances that are known to be genotoxic, there are even more that sit on the cusp. Some sources will tell you an oil is safe to use while pregnant, while other sources will tell you to avoid the same oil at all costs.

I'm not one to recommend something that could be harmful to an unborn child, so I think it's best to avoid (or at least severely restrict) your exposure to most essential oils while pregnant. The risks far outweigh the benefits when an unborn fetus is involved.

There are essential oils that are considered safe to use while pregnant. If you do decide you want to use these essential oils, always—and I mean always—consult with both your doctor and an aromatherapy professional before you do. There may be a very good reason why you should avoid using the oil(s) you're considering.

As far as using essential oils while breastfeeding goes, it's generally considered safe, as long as you're careful which oils you use. Make sure you're getting therapeutic grade essential oils from reputable sources and do your due diligence to make sure they're safe to use while nursing. Certain oils or components of the oils may pass through into your breast milk. If an oil contains something unsafe or that's a potential toxin or irritant, you're better off not using it.

There are a handful of essential oils that can help increase milk flow. The following essential oils are thought to improve the flow of milk:

- Basil oil (some sources say not to use this oil).
- Clary sage oil.
- Fennel oil.
- Grapeseed oil.

Consult with your doctor as to the proper dosage and technique to use, but typically a few drops added to a couple tablespoons of carrier oil is more than enough to get the milk flowing. Massage the oil into your breasts once a day. Wipe down the area where you massaged the oil in before breast feeding.

Essential Oil Blends

Essential oil blends are combinations of essential oils that have been blended for a specific purpose or to create a specific scent. There are literally thousands, if not tens of thousands, of blends on the market today, covering everything from athlete's foot to easing the effects of breathing conditions.

While you could buy your blends pre-mixed, that would mean missing out on half of the fun of aromatherapy. To me, the best part is mixing and matching the essential oils to create blends that have interesting and unique aromas and a potent combination of health benefits.

In order to understand how to blend essential oils, you're going to need to have at least a basic understanding of *notes*, which denote how strong of a scent the oil is going to have when blended. There are three basic types of notes:

- *Top notes* are the first notes you catch of whiff of when the fragrance reaches your nose. They're usually light notes that dissipate quickly. Top notes generally come from inexpensive oils.
- *Middle notes* are the softer notes that you smell once the top notes dissipate. Most essential oils are classified as middle notes.
- *Base notes* are heavier notes that take a while to come into their own and tend to linger around once they evolve. They're the stronger notes that stick around well after the top and middle notes have

disappeared. Essential oils that are considered top notes typically command a premium.

The following chart lists the note classifications of many of the essential oils used in blends today:

Top Notes	Middle Notes	Base Notes
Basil	African Bluegrass	Agarwood
Bergamot	Aljwain Seed	Amyris
Cajeput	Allspice	Angelica Root
Cinnamon	Amber	Cinnamon
Clary Sage	Ambrette Seed	Clove
Anise Oil	Armoise	Calamus
Bay	Balsam Peru	Cedarwood
Coriander	Bay Laurel	Cubeb
Calendula	Cardamom	Cypress
Cistus	Chamomile	Davana
Eucalyptus	Cypress	Erigeron
Grapefruit	Cocoa Absolute	Fennel
Galbanum	Cade	Frankincense
Garlic	Calendula	Ginger
Hyssop	White Camphor	Helichrysum
Hiba	Cananga	Harshingar
Lavender	Caraway	Oak Moss
Lemon	Carrot Seed	Patchouli
Lemongrass	Cassia	Sandalwood

Lime	Catnip	Spikenard
Mandarin	Celery Seed	Turmeric
Melissa	Cistus	Vetiver
Myrtle	Citronella	Ylang Ylang
Orange	Coffee	
Palo Santo	Cubeb	
Peppermint	Cumin	
Petitgrain	Dill Seed	
Rose	Douglas Fir	
Sage	Elemi	
Spearmint	Fennel	
Spruce	Geranium	
Tangerine	Galanga	
Vanilla	Goldenrod	
	Ginger Grass	
	Hyssop	
	Inula	
	Jasmine Absolute	
	Juniper Berry	
	Manuka	
	Marjoram	
	May Chang	
	Melissa	
	Mountain Savory	

	Myrrh	
	Neroli	
	Niaouli	
	Nutmeg	
	Oregano	
	Palmarosa	
	Parsley Seed	
	Pine	
	Ravensara	
	Rosemary	
	Rosewood	
	Tea Tree	
	Thyme	
	Wintergreen	
	Yarrow	
	Ylang Ylang	

You may notice some of the oils are in more than one column. This is because they are complex fragrances that feature scents that fall into more than one note classification. Combining these fragrances with others can be a bit tricky, but intricate blends with amazing fragrances can be created with a little practice.

You may also see other charts and resources that list these oils in different note categories. If there's one thing for certain about blending essential oils, it's that nothing's for certain. There's quite bit of discord when it comes to classifying oils. That's part to blame on the nuances between oils from different manufacturers and part the fact that no two people will smell something exactly alike.

Keep in mind that this chart is for general reference purposes only and essential oils of the same type can vary in fragrance from manufacturer to manufacturer. An oil that contains strong top notes when purchased at one manufacturer may have stronger middle notes when purchased at another. When in doubt, check with your supplier to see where the oils they sell should be classified—or just trust your nose. Your opinion is the only one that really matters when it comes to scent.

Ideally you want to blend your oils so they have a tantalizing top note that leads into a well-matched middle note that in turn gives way to a base note that lingers around for a while. How you accomplish this is up to you. There are formulas in books and online that give guidelines as to what percentage of each type of note you should use, but I've found that these guidelines are rarely strictly adhered to. Use what you need to use to give your blends and products the scent that you want them to have, not what someone else tells you to use. Rules are made to be broken and most blends I've seen are only loosely based on any ruleset.

You also need to keep in mind the fact that even though an oil may be classified as a certain note, the strength of that oil may be able to overpower the rest of your blend if you use it at too high of a concentration. If you don't want strong-scented oils to overpower your blends, then you should only use a drop or two of the stronger oils and add more of the weaker oils to balance them out.

Aromatic Blends

Are you ready to start blending essential oils and creating your own recipes, but not quite sure where to start? The following recipes are a great start into the world of essential oils. Use therapeutic grade essential oils in all of your blends for best results.

Always start off with small amounts of oil in your blends and test them in a small area for a reaction before moving up to the amount of oil indicated in the recipe. You don't want to apply an oil blend or product and find out you're allergic to it after you've applied it to your entire body.

These blends can be used for a number of purposes. They can be added to products, diffused and mixed with carrier oil and applied topically. Make sure you test them in smaller amounts first to make sure they aren't going to cause problems. These blends should not be applied to the skin at full strength.

If you plan on diffusing your oil blend, multiply the recipe by 5, blend the oils and use 10 to 15 drops of the blend in the diffuser.

Keep in mind that these aren't the only blends that exist. This list is just to get you started and show you what's popular. You can mix and match essential oils with various properties to create healthy blends with all sorts of fragrances and therapeutic qualities.

Acne

Dilute this blend with carrier oil and apply topically.

4 drops lavender

3 drops tea tree

1 drop geranium

Calming #1

2 drops bergamot

3 drops lavender

2 drops sandalwood

Calming #2

1 drop clary sage

2 drops lavender

2 drops rose

1 drop vetiver

Cold and Flu #1

1 drop eucalyptus

2 drops lemon

2 drop rosemary

Cold and Flu #2

1 drop tea tree

2 drops lemon

2 drop rosemary

Cold and Flu #3

2 drops cinnamon

2 drops pine

2 drops rosemary

Congestion #1

2 drops chamomile

3 drops eucalyptus

1 drop anise

3 drops lemon

Congestion #2

2 drops eucalyptus

2 drops peppermint

2 drops cedarwood

Dandruff

Dilute this oil with carrier oil and apply to scalp. Always test in a small area first.

2 drops basil

2 drops cypress

1 drop lemon

1 drop patchouli

2 drops tea tree

Energy #1

2 drops ginger

1 drop grapefruit

1 drop bergamot

Energy #2

2 drops lemon

1 drop grapefruit

2 drops peppermint

Energy #3

3 drops lemon

3 drops rosemary

Focus #1

2 drops cypress

1 drop rosemary

1 drop peppermint

Focus #2

1 drop basil

2 drops cypress

2 drops lemon

Happiness #1

2 drops grapefruit

1 drop rose

2 drops sandalwood

Happiness #2

3 drops lemon

3 drops grapefruit

2 drops ylang ylang

Happiness #3

2 drops geranium

1 drop frankincense

2 drops neroli

Happiness #4

2 drops bergamot

2 drops jasmine

1 drop rose

1 drop sandalwood

Happiness #5

2 drops basil

1 drop rose

1 drop geranium

1 drop Melissa

2 drops sandalwood

Happiness #6

2 drops lavender

1 drop lemon

1 drop orange

1 drop peppermint

2 drops ylang ylang

Happy Hair

4 drops lavender oil

4 drops lemon oil

5 drops tea tree oil

Inflammation

Never apply this oil at full strength. It needs to be diluted heavily before application.

2 drops clove bud

2 drops peppermint

Insect Repellent

Do not apply this oil topically!

3 drops citronella

2 drops cedarwood

2 drops eucalyptus

2 drops tea tree oil

2 drops patchouli

Odor Remover #1

3 drops lavender

1 drop orange

1 drop lemon

1 drop lime

2 drops nutmeg

Odor Remover #2

2 drops bergamot

2 drops cinnamon

2 drops orange

1 drop sage

Odor Remover #3

2 drops cinnamon

3 drops lime

2 drops jasmine

2 drops orange

Odor Remover #4

2 drops bergamot

1 drop lemon

1 drop lime

2 drops ylang ylang

Odor Remover #5

3 drops lemon

2 drops patchouli

2 drops thyme

Sleepy Time #1

3 drops lavender

2 drops marjoram

2 drops Roman chamomile

1 drop ylang ylang

Sleepy Time #2

2 drops bergamot

2 drops clary sage

2 drops lavender

3 drops Roman chamomile

Sleepy Time #3

2 drops basil

1 drop neroli

2 drops Roman chamomile

Stress Relief #1

3 drops bergamot

1 drop rose

2 drops sandalwood

Stress Relief #2

2 drops clary sage

2 drops lavender

1 drop patchouli

1 drop vetiver

Stress Relief #3

2 drops bergamot

4 drops geranium

2 drops lavender

4 drops ylang ylang

Stress Relief #4

2 drops clary sage

2 drops elemi

2 drops frankincense

2 drops lavender

2 drops ylang ylang

Bonus Recipe: Lavender-Honey Bath Melts

This recipe is from one of my other books: "How to Make Bath Melts and Bombs." Click on the link below to find this book on Amazon.com:

http://www.amazon.com/dp/B00AMV8ZWM

If you aren't familiar with bath melts, you don't know what you're missing. You throw one in the tub and it disperses oil and butter throughout the tub, leaving you smelling and feeling great.

Ingredients:

10 ounces cocoa butter

2 ounces Shea butter

.4 ounces honey

20 drops lavender essential oil

1 ounce dried lavender flowers

Directions:

1. Melt cocoa butter and Shea butter in a double broiler.
2. Stir in the honey.
3. Remove from heat and let cool for a few minutes until it starts to thicken. Continue stirring every once in a while to keep powdered oats from settling.
4. Add the lavender essential oil and the dried lavender flowers and stir until evenly distributed.
5. Pour into a mold and store in a cool, dry place until the melts set. You can place the mold in the refrigerator to speed up the process.

Use:

Toss the bath melt in the tub while it's filling. It will melt and disperse oil and butter throughout the tub. Hop in the tub and enjoy! The butter and oil will rise to the top and will leave a light coating of beneficial oil and butter on your skin. You'll smell great and feel good for the rest of the day.

The End of the Book, the Beginning of Your Journey

So you've reached the end of the book. I hope you learned a lot about essential oils and their many uses. I also hope that this book is the catalyst for those of you who aren't already using these oils to at least give them a try.

They really are that powerful. In fact, many people credit essential oils as having changed their life and helped them manage and even treat a number of illnesses and ailments. I've used them myself for a number of purposed.

Don't let reaching the end of this book be the end of your journey into the world of essential oils. Instead, use it as the jumping off point for further research and learning. You can thank me later.

<barcode>|||||| ||| | ||||||| ||||| ||||||| |||| ||||||| ||| ||</barcode>

3992540R00184

Printed in Great Britain
by Amazon.co.uk, Ltd.,
Marston Gate.